MONICA BRANT'S

Secrets to Staying Fit & Loving Life!

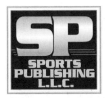

SP
SPORTS PUBLISHING
L.L.C.

www.SportsPublishingLLC.com

ISBN: 1-59670-068-8

All cover and interior photos by Robert Reiff/www.magiclight.com, unless noted otherwise.

Publishers: Peter L. Bannon and Joseph J. Bannon Sr.
Senior managing editor: Susan M. Moyer
Acquisitions editor: Dean Miller
Developmental editor: Erin Linden-Levy
Art director: K. Jeffrey Higgerson
Cover/dust jacket design: Joseph Brumleve
Interior layout: Heidi Norsen
Imaging: Heidi Norsen
Media and promotions managers: Jonathan Patterson (regional),
     Randy Fouts (national), Maurey Williamson (print)

Printed in the United States of America

Sports Publishing L.L.C.
804 North Neil Street
Champaign, IL 61820

Phone: 1-877-424-2665
Fax: 217-363-2073

Dedication

First and foremost, this book is dedicated
to my Savior, Jesus Christ.
Without His guidance, wisdom in His Word,
and love, I would not be in my
"favorite place in life" as I am now.

Secondly, this book is dedicated to all the
fans and friends whom I have met
and made around the world who have
given me both inspiration and support for
the last 10 years of my career. Thanks for
all your thoughts and words along
the way. You are all very appreciated!

Table of *Contents*

Medical Note:

This book should not be substituted for medical advice. If you're pregnant, recovering from an injury or suffering from any health condition, check with your physician for guidelines.

Foreword

By Marla Duncan

My love of weight lifting began when I was 16 years old and I decided that the girls' jazzercise class was not as fun or challenging as the boys' weight-lifting class! Upon this realization I asked my PE teacher if I could switch classes. Little did I know that changing my PE class would also begin changing my future.

As I continued to lift weights throughout high school my body became curvy and muscular. In order to showcase all my hard work, in 1983 I began swimsuit modeling and participated in calendar girl pageants, beauty pageants and bikini competitions. Even though I won many contests, I was always labeled the "muscular one" and did not necessarily fit in with the current ideal for women's bodies.

In 1989, I discovered a new and exciting opportunity, created for women just like me. It was exactly what I was looking for—the dawn of a new athlete the world had never seen before: the fitness competitor. I eagerly joined this new sport and won a major competition in 1990, the Ms. Fitness USA contest. Over the next few years, the fitness industry grew and a large fan base developed. Monica Brant was one of the main competitors to emerge as the industry evolved through the years.

I would later discover that I was an inspiration for Monica as she began her career in Fitness. She cut my photos out of a fitness magazine and taped them to her mirror for inspiration! What a great feeling to know that, in the past 15 years, I have been a positive influence and role model, not just to Monica, but to others as well. After all, my passion has always been to help others achieve their personal fitness goals.

When I first met Monica in 1995 she spoke of her admiration for my accomplishments and told me that she hoped to follow in my footsteps in the fitness and health industry. Needless to say I was flattered; that, in my humble opinion, is the highest form of gratification anyone can receive.

Over the past decade, Monica's dedication and professionalism have enabled her to exceed my accomplishments, and she has created a legacy of her very own.

In *Monica Brant's Secrets to Staying Fit & Loving Life!* Monica demonstrates her leadership ability and educates readers

(continued on page viii)

about the benefits of a healthy lifestyle. She presents an eating regimen and the foundational training principles in a simple and basic format that's fun and motivational!

After reading *Monica Brant's Secrets to Staying Fit & Loving Life!*, I hope you will absorb the valuable information you have just read and apply it to YOUR life! There is never a better time to get started than RIGHT NOW!

Like Monica, this book is real, down to earth and believable! It has been quite an honor to be a part of its development and success.

Work hard, stay determined and make your dreams come true!

Marla Duncan
Ms. Fitness USA, 1990
Wife and mother of
two darling boys,
Wyatt and Kelson

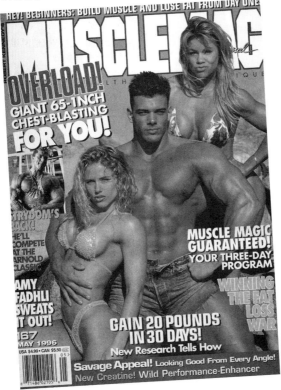

Monica Brant (left), Frank Sepe (middle) and Marla Duncan (right). *MuscleMag International* magazine, May 1996.
Used with permission.

Acknowledgments

I would like to take this opportunity to thank some people and companies for their help and support throughout this book project. Without each of you, I would still be "bookless"!

My husband, Scott, for all his patience with me while I typed endlessly—thanks, my "10," for giving me the confidence to move forward with this project!

Bradford Licensing Associates—thanks for believing in me and helping secure an awesome publishing company. Visit them on the web at www.bradfordlicensing.com.

Sports Publishing L.L.C. for all their support and patience while I was traveling and having to push the book deadline back—sorry! They can be found on the web at www.sportspublishingllc.com.

My mom, Patti—thanks for the constant encouragement. You are an amazing mom; I hope I can be the same someday!

Robert Reiff—thank you for taking some awesome shots for the book (and over the last 10-plus years) and for being such a great friend, always ready with helpful advice. Robert's website can be found at www.magiclight.com.

Beth Saltz, for editing this book and giving me the encouragement to actually do one—you believed in me from the get-go. It took me some time to get moving, huh? Congrats on being a new mommy—Zoe is beautiful!

Nancy Jambazian, for making sure my hair and makeup were just right—you are a very talented lady. Love you lots!

Kim Oddo, for spending the day with us on our shoot and making sure my form was perfect—good eye! Also, thanks for the years of friendship and support on the good ol' diet. I'm glad to have spent my last years competing with you on my team. You are the best! Visit Kim online at www.bodybyo.com.

(continued on page x)

Weider Publications—thank you for allowing me to snoop through all the photos that were taken of me for your company over the last 10-plus years (and to publish a few!). You can find Weider online at www.muscleandfitness.com and www.muscleandfitnesshers.com.

Robert Kennedy and Kerrie Lee Brown, for all the support through *Oxygen* and *MuscleMag International* magazines—I am so thankful for the encouragement and press you have given me. Keep up the fantastic work on the magazines! Find both magazines on the web at www.emusclemag.com and www.oxygenmag.com.

Margo Rombough—thanks for the incredible styling and for coming through at the last minute for me!

A special thank you to Elisabetta Rogiani for lending her beautiful fitness clothing for the cover and training shots. Be sure to watch for her incredible line on celebrities everywhere! You can find her clothing online at www.rogiani.com.

Photographer Cory Sorensen—thank you for allowing me to use your photos! Awesome work!

Photographer Irv Gelb—thanks for allowing me to use your photos, too! We have a long history of great shooting together.

Versa Gripps, the best straps ever—thanks for helping me keep my grip! Check them out at www.versagripps.com.

MONICA BRANT'S

Secrets to Staying Fit & Loving Life!

MY STORY

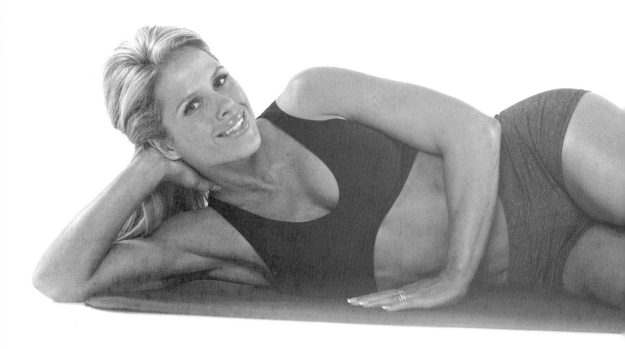

Jumping
into Fitness

Well, here goes my tale. I plan to do my best to share my background and experiences with you in hopes that they will give you some smiles and inspiration in your own walk of life! If you do not immediately know who I am, please take a few minutes and read my introduction to find out for yourself why I have been compelled to write this book and why it might help you grow in your own personal goals.

Even though I am certified through the International Sports Sciences Association (ISSA), I must humbly admit that I am not an expert in the field of nutrition or training. What I do have is over 10 years of experience in the fitness industry, as well as knowledge from surrounding myself with educated trainers and nutritionists. It took me many years to actually gain the courage to write this book and feel capable of having enough valuable information to share with you.

After many fans asked me to write a book, I gained some momentum and started this project. As in beginning a new training program, *starting* was the hardest part. I had never written this much in one sitting and I have renewed appreciation for authors now. Writing a short article or answering "Q&As" is nothing compared to writing a book—it has been quite an experience for me.

It is my heart's desire that by reading this book you will learn something, have some fun and, most importantly, understand that you are not alone in your struggles and challenges regarding living a healthy and fit life.

My fitness story began in early 1991 when I first saw a photo of a national fitness competition winner in a fitness magazine. I was in awe of her physique and I felt compelled to find out more about her and the contest. The winner I admired was Marla Duncan, and the contest was the 1990 Fitness USA Nationals. I immediately ordered the contest video and basically waited by the mailbox to receive it. I was excited, to say the least.

At this same time I had just met a trainer from a local gym and began serious training, committed to making my workouts a priority four days a week. Since we were both young and mostly uneducated in the gym, I was training with heavy weights on all of my body parts. I do not believe my friend knew any better, and he was simply training me as he would himself. Keeping track of my workouts (weights, sets, reps) was important, and I could see a definite increase in the weight I was lifting. I am a very strong girl! This type of workout may not have been ideal, but it was a good start, and I do not feel it hindered or hurt me in any way whatsoever.

Finally the fitness competition video arrived and I studied it with family and friends to see if it was something I should participate in. At this time I had been competing in some bikini contests in and around San Antonio and felt that fitness competition would be a nice step up from local contests.

For those of you unfamiliar with fitness competitions, the format varies, but you're essentially judged on the shape and condition of your physique, along with different rounds such as a gymnastics/dance-based routine, a series of mandatory strength/conditioning movements, a speaking round and/or an obstacle course. The format varies by show and changes as promoters experiment with new ideas.

The competitions I began doing were comprised of three rounds: physique, fitness routine, and a poise round. These seemed a bit intimidating, as I was uncomfortable speaking in front of people and inexperienced for the fitness routine. (Thankfully, back in the early '90s the routines were not as advanced as today's fitness routines—which sometimes look like gymnastics competitions.) However, I was not going to let these issues stop me from pursuing the event, so I located a choreographer and a pageant consultant for the poise round.

The poise round was judged on the ability to walk in heels, wearing a gown, and explain your "philosophy of fitness." I definitely had to spend some time learning the art of speaking in front of an audience, and at any given family function, my family would have me stand up in front of them and recite my speech. I had to work hard to gain confidence and learn to present myself. The pageant instructor was of great help, and I quickly learned to be more graceful and fluid.

Regarding the routine round, I found it difficult (and quite amusing) to learn a routine since I had no prior training in dance, gymnastics or even in aerobics classes. The "choreographer" I hired happened to be an instructor at my gym and he insisted I take his dance/step class to become familiar with some moves as well as gain some timing and rhythm. I

remember trying to learn the "Roger Rabbit" dance step and the "Grapevine." I never mastered the "Roger Rabbit," but I believe I have the "Grapevine" down after all these years!

Finally, (after many funny and frustrating moments) we arranged a simple routine for my first show, which was in the fall of 1991—just about six months after I decided to compete in Fitness. To this day the show was a blur to me, but I somehow made it through a routine (probably not the actual routine) and also did well enough in the poise round to land first place. Okay, so there were only two of us in the show, but no matter...it was a win and I was hooked.

The Early Years

Allow me to take a step back in time and share my background with you, so you can understand what brought me to the fitness stage. I grew up in the hill country outside of San Antonio, Texas, in a small town called Castroville. Since the age of five, I was accustomed to riding and showing horses. This came naturally since my mom trained horses and gave riding lessons at our horse ranch.

I continued to show horses through my school years and I developed a desire to try out for cheerleading in high school. However, the rules of cheerleading stipulated that I first must spend one year in pep squad prior to tryouts. During that year, I watched the other cheerleaders,

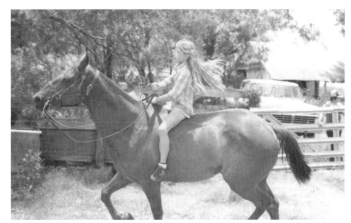

keeping notes on the tricks they would perform, such as back handsprings, aerials, and different types of jumps. I would go home almost every day after school and practice these tricks on our home trampoline. Once I could do them on the trampoline I was motivated to try the moves on the ground. Well, I muscled my way through back handsprings, aerials, back tucks, front flips, front handsprings, and all kinds of jumps. Of course my technique was mostly off, but I still managed to fly through the air and land on my feet. I was sure this was going to land me a position on the cheerleading team the following year.

Following the pep squad year, my mom and I had a heart-to-heart discussion about cheerleading. She made it clear that I could either do cheerleading or continue to show my horses, but not both—the expense would be too much. The choice was not hard to make; I loved the horse industry and loved the showing events I had grown up doing each year. So that was the end of my experience in cheerleading, but those tricks I taught myself ended up being the tricks I used for my early fitness competition routines.

In high school I ran track and played volleyball. (Incidentally, my 1,600-meter relay team won the 1986 Texas State Championship. I ran the second leg.) I'd alternate between track meets and volleyball games at school and then ride and train horses after school and during the summer. Some family friends actually gave me the opportunity to earn $20 per hour training their horses and giving riding lessons. Doing something I loved—riding horses—was a great way to learn to work. In addition to training other people's horses and giving riding lessons, I continued with the daily care of my own horses to prepare them for the summer show circuit.

Looking back, I know that I learned so much about discipline, dedication and hard work through those early years. I was given quite a big responsibility with the horses that were brought to our barn. I had to keep very clear notes as to what I did each day with the horses I had in my care and what progress they were or were not making. Not once did I feel incapable of teaching the horses to do certain things, and I'll never forget being the first to ride the last horse that was born on our property. The experiences definitely prepared me for the type of dedication I have to have today to endure the rigors of my job. Even back then I believe God had certain lessons for me to learn about goals.

I believe those early-developed character qualities (along with my Christian faith) are the main reasons I have been able to endure this fitness sport and turn it into a career.

Taking the
Stage

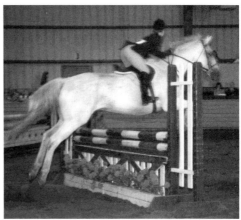

Now let's return to my first show and to the "philosophy of fitness" I developed. I remember that my statement centered on hard work, dedication to a healthy lifestyle, and admiration for the two women who were (and are to this day!) my role models: my grandma and my mom. Both of these women taught me the fundamentals of discipline and follow-through in making decisions and setting goals.

Having won my first contest in August 1991, I was then qualified to compete in the Ms. National Fitness USA competition that was scheduled for later that year in Las Vegas, Nevada. (Imagine back then if I knew that I would still be competing in Las Vegas throughout 2005—14 years later!) At Nationals, even though I was scared to death, I came in 14th out of about 30 girls. I felt dizzy and had a migraine the entire show, so I'm not sure how I even placed that high.

For some reason, after the national show I decided Fitness was just not for me. I quit training at the gym and probably gained some weight from my lack of exercise during 1992. I believe I was still trying to figure out who I was and what I wanted to do with my life. My ultimate dream of being an equestrian rider in the Olympics seemed to be an entire lifetime away, so I enrolled at San Antonio College (SAC), worked as a waitress and modeled for Budweiser Brewery as a "Bud" girl. I continued to earn extra money, entering bikini contests in the local nightclubs as

As I read the draft of Monica's book, I am in awe of the unfolding of her life! Not only am I proud of what she has accomplished, I am so very pleased with how she has dedicated her life to our Savior, Jesus Christ. When Monica was 16, I prayed, asking God what name He would give her as He had renamed others in scripture. I was impressed as He gently said she is "My Loving Testimony." Monica has certainly lived up to this calling and continues to fulfill it daily in all the lives that she touches in small or great ways. She positioned herself early on to allow God to be in control of the circumstances of her life in order that He could bring forth the best opportunities for her.

Those Monica has blessed with love and counsel are too numerous to count. I join in with the thousands of people of all ages who find Monica to be an inspiration and encouragement. Her purpose and desire is to assist others to focus on their gifts and strengths and then to allow God's help to develop the weaker areas of concern, not just physically, but mentally, emotionally and spiritually. This is how she lives her own life, so she passionately imparts it to others as well.

Monica leads with her heart. This book is a product of her heart.

I am delighted to be Monica's mom,
Patti

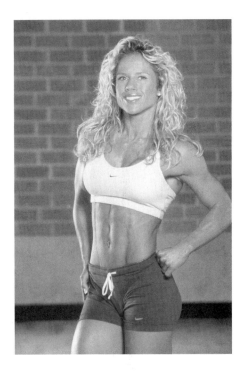

life at that time, but I do feel He made good out of any wrong choices I may have made. God has taken what I chose to do in the past and made it useful today. I know that my heart is set on God and that some of my decisions may not have been His choice, but He has used those exact things to refine me and to give me confidence. For example, I gained poise, confidence, and understanding from entering all those bikini contests; and I learned to save and spend my money wisely.

Back to the
Fitness
story...

well as different "leg and tan" contests. I remember being disciplined with the money I earned and would add it to my savings account each time I competed.

Speaking of discipline and dedication, I am sure some of you may be thinking, "How could a Christian do these kinds of contests with a clear conscience?" I was raised in a Christian home and attended church throughout my junior high and high school years. After graduating from high school I still attended church and knew where my heart was regarding my faith and relationship with God. Even though I am sure God was not necessarily in favor of me entering all those bikini contests, I truly believe He turned me towards the lifestyle in which I am now involved. Had I not gained confidence being onstage in those bikini contests, I may not ever have felt capable of competing in Fitness. I do believe that my choices may not have always been the best ones, or perhaps not in God's will for my

As I said, I quit competing after the 1991 Nationals. I don't have a real reason for quitting; it was probably mostly due to being young and not yet having a real visualization of the future. I did not know anyone involved in the fitness business and needed to concentrate on the other things going on in my life. In the spring of 1993, a bodybuilding competitor I knew asked me why I wasn't competing in Fitness; he thought I had the physique for it. I then started "reconnecting" with Fitness and thinking about taking the stage once again.

So, I resumed weight training in 1993 and decided to compete again. This time I sought the help of the San Antonio Spurs Silverdancers coach. She was a huge help to me, and I learned many exciting moves from her. I also incorporated those self-taught gymnastics that I learned on the trampoline at home those many years ago. We developed a cute routine, which I actually remembered onstage.

I entered the Texas USA semifinals in September 1993 and placed sixth—disappointing to me. Since I did not place in the top few spots, I was not qualified for the next step, Nationals. My qualifying show ended up being a disaster. Not only did I come in *one place* behind qualifying for Nationals, my rented gown was stolen from the dressing room while I was onstage. That was a very expensive contest, since I had to pay for the dress.

During late 1993 I went with a girlfriend to see another friend of ours compete in a bodybuilding competition in Tijuana, Mexico. He introduced me to John Parillo, who in turned introduced me to two very nice gentlemen, Ralph DeHaan and Steve Wennerstrom, all of whom were strongly involved in the fitness industry.

All three of these men encouraged me to continue in my fitness competitions and welcomed me to take some test shots if I made it to California.

That was in December, and by June of 1994 I had prepared for a competition in Venice, California. I knew that competing with the California girls would be a big challenge. This time around I had a team of supporters going with me—who could resist going to California during the summer? The competition was held at Venice High School, and lo and behold I placed an amazing *first*. Wow—I couldn't believe it! I was thrilled.

After the competition, my best friend and I drove to San Diego and I had my first official photo shoot for the fitness industry with Ralph DeHaan, who was then a Weider photographer. After my shoot, Ralph suggested we stay a second day and do a "test" shoot with the winner of the USA National Bodybuilding Competition, Dennis Newman. Ralph was scheduled to photograph Dennis the following day. Of course my girlfriend and I stayed, and I did the shoot with no expectations of it ending up anywhere.

I went home with such enthusiasm that I decided right away to prepare for Fitness Nationals to be held once again in Vegas later that year. That show was not very memorable, mostly because I ended up getting another migraine headache—probably from too much stress and too little food. I remember feeling like I was going to pass out during the physique round and barely getting through my routine. This time around I came in ninth, a slight step up from the previous national-level show I did. With this contest under my belt for the year, I started to think about getting ready for the Fitness USA Nationals in Buena Park, California, which was not until February 1995.

Moving Up and Out

While I was home preparing for the show I got one of the most exciting calls ever. The photographer, Ralph DeHaan, called, and all I remember from his mes-

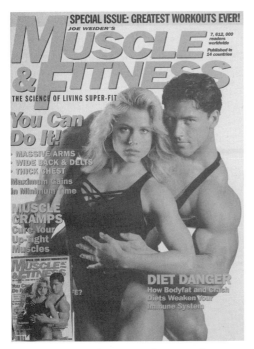

This was my very first cover of a national magazine! This issue was on newsstands in November 1994, but the photo was taken in June that same year. The male bodybuilder is Dennis Newman, 1994 USA Overall Champion. Used with permission.

sage on my machine was "Hi, cover girl!" It seemed unreal to me, but I had actually made the cover of the prestigious *Muscle & Fitness* magazine for November 1994.

Knowing I had a cover coming out made me even more focused and excited to prepare for the next show. I continued to train and practice with all the intensity I could muster. When the day finally came for me to leave for the competition I could barely sit still. I had many good friends with me to cheer me on, and of course my family came out. My dad still complains about having to carry my bag, which was filled with cans of tuna and dumbbells. Ha! I must have imagined California did not have tuna or dumbbells!

Upon arrival I realized it was going to be a huge show—the promoters had a film crew taping the event for television. We had to learn a short routine for the opening and then had to synchronize with over 150 girls for the rest of the show. I had no idea that there would be so much work involved in the production; it was quite overwhelming.

If coming in ninth in this event was not enough, I met Jan Tana, who is a leader in the fitness industry and runs her own yearly competitions. She was there sponsoring another athlete and I decided to give her one of my composite photo cards. (Knowing I was going to be meeting many different people, I was prepared and had made comp cards prior to the show.) This opened the door for me to be invited to compete in Jan Tana's first Pro Fitness show in July 1995.

At this time I was debating a move to California. I felt compelled to move, even though I did not have any idea what I would do for income. Being the independent girl that I am, I made the decision to go for it and just see what I could do in California.

Arriving in sunny Los Angeles was scary, but exciting, for me. The only people I knew in the area were my roommate, who traveled all the time, and Ralph, the photographer in San Diego. Thankfully I was not afraid of being alone, and I learned my way around quickly. Making my way to the gym was a priority, and I ended up at Gold's Gym, Redondo Beach. It was now the end of April 1995 and since I was planning to compete at the Jan Tana Pro Fitness Classic at the end of July, I had to get busy finding a choreographer.

I met a wonderfully talented choreographer, Lisa Nunziella-Hockley, who helped me gain the confidence and skills I needed to compete at the next level. As well as being a professional dancer for movies, she also instructed a dance class at Gold's Gym, Venice. I learned how to do a split leap, high kick, strength moves

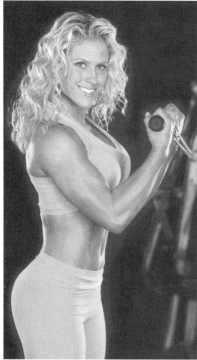

and some cool dance moves. I thoroughly enjoyed my training and felt like we put together a fantastic routine—of course I felt it was one of my fitness career's best. I ended up winning the Jan Tana Pro Fitness contest that summer and was invited to the very first International Federation of Bodybuilding (IFBB) Fitness Olympia later that same year. What an amazing first year!

Lisa coached me for many years, but in 1997 I decided I needed to add to my skills by taking private gymnastic lessons. My coach and I worked on new moves and I re-learned my homemade tumbling—finally learning proper techniques and saving my body from damage. It was crazy...I could do a flip, but not a proper cartwheel. I found that gymnastics was very tough on the body and quite challenging—especially at my age (late 20s at the time).

I continued to compete in the IFBB Pro Fitness Circuit, and in November 1998 I won the prestigious Fitness Olympia competition, which was held in Nice, France. It is hard to believe I made it so far with my limited dance and gymnastics background. It just goes to show that with determination and dedication, one can accomplish any goal.

In 1999 I had a change of heart and decided that I'd had enough of fitness competitions. Even though I enjoyed the challenge of preparing for competitions, I lacked the motivation to continue with the grueling gymnastics training that was increasing with each contest I entered.

Although I retired from fitness competitions, I stayed very involved with the fitness business. I continued to do photo shoots for various fitness magazines and made appearances all over the world—throughout the U.S., as well as Canada, Germany, Italy, Austria, Japan, Malaysia, Mexico, St. Marten, Bahamas, Jamaica, Australia, South Africa, Brazil, and Argentina. In addition, I continued with my representation agreement with the top international supplement company, Universal Nutrition.

In January 2003, the first invitational Pro Figure competition was held in conjunction with the already popular Arnold Classic Bodybuilding & Fitness Competition. I was invited to compete and felt a strong conviction to once again step onto the stage. Figure competitions are basically fitness competitions without the routine; therefore, no gymnastics are required. Since that first figure competition, I have continued to compete and place in the top two or three for each figure show. I have enjoyed being back on stage and feel very thankful to be able to compete successfully after all these years.

I can definitely admit that making a career out of the fitness industry has been quite a learning experience. Never in a million years did I dream I would be honored with over 100 national and international magazine covers or that fans would ask me for autographs. That still blows my mind!

Looking back, I am positive that learning to work hard and spend wisely as a teenager made it possible to carve out a spot for myself in the fitness industry and make a living from the sport. Of course, along with my hard work and dedication, I also continue to ask God to keep opening and closing doors for me, keeping me in His will for my future. It has been quite an honor to be able to meet so many wonderful people throughout the world and be a source of inspiration to others as they follow their dreams and goals!

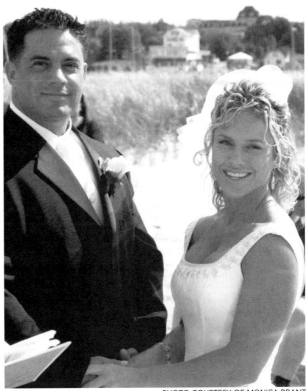

PHOTO COURTESY OF MONICA BRANT

Thankfully, God is still opening doors for me and helping me make wise decisions for my future, such as new and fun events like the Monica Brant Fitness Classic (we celebrated our sixth event in 2005) and the F.E.M. Camps, where I can give back to the new athletes in the sport by providing direction and guidance in the fitness industry, as well as advice regarding competing, training, modeling, and motivation.

Another answered prayer is my marriage to a wonderful man named Scott Peckham. After being in California for 10 years, I'm ready for my next stage of life, as Scott and I are planning to move to Austin, Texas. Scott and I are a great team, and we are looking forward to the opportunities in our future. Even though I am married and will hopefully one day have kids, you can guarantee that I'll continue to do everything in my power to inspire and motivate others to live healthy lifestyles!

Thank you for taking the time to read my little bit of history. I hope it gives you inspiration to tackle your own dreams and goals. There is no time like the present to start...please read on to find out how simple it can really be!

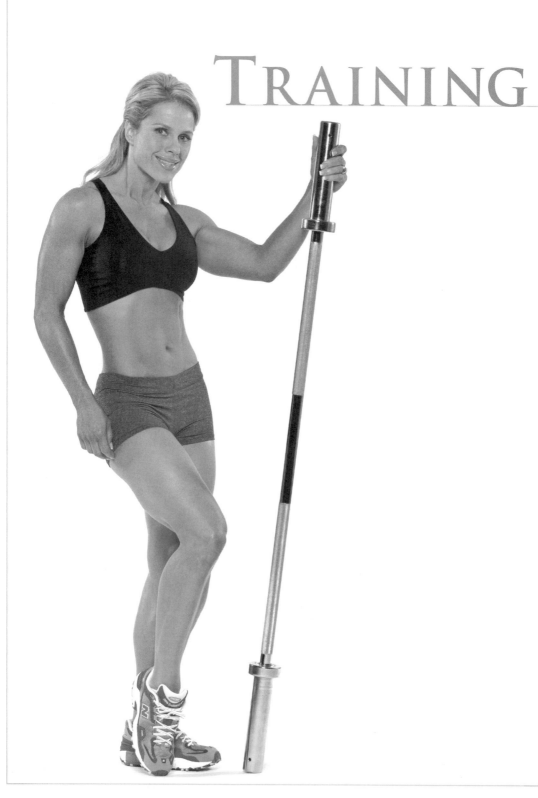

TRAINING

Why 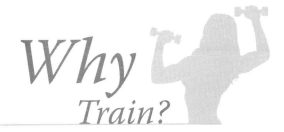 *Train?*

For many years I have been encouraging women who want to better their physiques to train with weights, but still I get the question about becoming "built like a man." One would think that with all the ads for fitness centers and the hundreds of gyms you see in every city, women would run to the gym like ducks to water in order to acquire (or keep) curvy shapes and good health. Still, unfortunately, I think many women shy away from weight training because of what they think might happen to their ladylike figures.

I promise, in all my years of fitness, I have never seen a woman "bulk up" with too much muscle from a *normal* weight-training regimen.

So back to the question at hand: "Why train?"

Well, my fitness friends, there are many reasons to train with weights, but for me the most exciting reason is to have a fit and healthy physique now and, more importantly, later in life.

That is reason enough for me to head to the gym a few times a week! Just in case that is not enough to entice you to start a weight-training program, allow me to share some other benefits of weight training, including:

- *Burning fat (I believe this is the best one)*
- *Building muscles, which will produce stronger, denser bones (especially important to prevent osteoporosis)*
- *Increasing flexibility in your overall movements*
- *Providing more energy for other activities, even if it is just getting through a hectic work day (think about all those great little endorphins that come out to play and energize you when you weight train—they will help you feel more confident and relaxed all day long)*
- *Reducing cravings for sweets by balancing emotional ups and downs*
- *Improving metabolic markers (like insulin) that may help you prevent or manage diseases such as diabetes*
- *Meeting great people in the gym (maybe your future soul mate)*

Besides weight training, a comprehensive program will also include cardiovascular exercise, rest, and proper nutrition to help shape/reshape your body and provide you with a longer, healthier, and happier life. Let's take a look at some of the benefits that exercise can have on a body:

- *Alleviating back aches (your core will become stronger and will help you stay in alignment)*
- *Helping/preventing depression*
- *Relieving headaches*
- *Helping to prevent heart disease and even cancer*

I feel it is safe to say that if exercise could be encapsulated in a pill, it would be the most widely prescribed drug in the world!

Let's move on with setting goals that will provide you with a road map for training, along with lots of motivation to keep you going strong. Now that I have your attention, let's get to the details of setting up your training program.

Setting Goals
for Reshaping
Your Physique

I firmly believe that everyone should evaluate their physiques with an experienced friend, relative, or personal trainer to determine what steps should be taken to reach their ultimate goals. In my opinion, almost all women need a stronger back and broader shoulders. Of course there are exceptions to this; some women are born with beautiful, shapely upper bodies. However, those of us (that includes me!) missing this genetic trait need to concentrate on our "V" taper by lifting slightly heavier weights to develop a wider back and rounder shoulder caps for the broad-shouldered look.

Remember when women's jackets and tops contained shoulder pads? This was to give the illusion of the "V" taper, which ultimately makes the waist appear smaller. That should be music to any woman's ear!

For those of you who already have a natural "V" taper, perhaps your legs need more work? In that case, you would alter your training program to lift heavier weights for legs and train your upper body with less weight but more sets.

It may be hard for some women to see where their body lines fall if they are carrying more body fat (don't feel bad, as this comes naturally for women). If this is the case, I strongly encourage concentrating on nutrition while you do a beginner's workout plan. You will lose some fat to see what shape you really have—some people never knew that they had shapely legs or abdominals. How exciting! Think of it like *slowly* unwrapping a present to prolong the excitement of discovering what is beneath the wrapping. My brother used to do this at Christmas every year—he would save all his presents and then insist that everyone watch him while he unwrapped his gifts slowly!

Okay, enough history; back to the goal setting. The following ideas are basic stuff, but we all need some reminders at times.

After contemplating your body structure, let me suggest writing down your long- and short-term goals. While a long-term goal could be a year or more into the future, short-term goals can range from days to weeks to months. Just as writing down your plans for the day in a calendar helps you focus on exactly what needs to be accomplished, writing down your goals will also help you think about where you want to see your physique someday.

Of course I suggest that you be realistic, too. It is okay to dream of being 9-12% body fat, as a top athlete will be, but if you are currently at 30% body fat it will take a lot of perseverance, work, and patience to get down to even 20%!

I suggest setting short-term goals for different timelines. Your goal for this week might be to get to the gym on Monday, Wednesday, and Friday. Your monthly goal may be to get to the gym 12 times and to do some cardio outdoors another five times. Other goals might be to drop 1-5% body fat in two months, or to lose one pound a week.

Set some realistic goals and concentrate on making those happen. You will be encouraged when you achieve your first goal, and then you can ride that wave of encouragement to your next goal and so on.

After putting your goals down on paper, you will need to arrange your routine, targeting the entire body, to effectively reduce body fat and strengthen your muscles. Keep in mind, this means making a commitment to yourself (and your routine) for six to eight weeks to start seeing improvements and reaping the benefits of training. You must have discipline and dedication to the training program; especially if training is new to you, that may be the hardest part. I am sure most of you will see improvements in less time, but I like to tell everyone to wait a bit longer, because by the fourth or fifth week you are usually hooked on training and have enthusiasm to continue. (Pretty sneaky, huh?)

One of the best ways I have found to keep your commitment to train, especially for "newbies," is to hire a professional personal trainer. A personal trainer will help you learn your way around the gym in a shorter period of time. A trainer will also help you learn proper form, preventing injuries that will keep you out of the gym and that much farther away from attaining your goals. You will also find that a personal trainer is someone to whom you are accountable. After all, you will be paying for his or her services and most people do not want to waste hard-earned money.

I have hired many different trainers over the years and have learned a variety of exercises that I can fall back on when I am in the gym. If you do hire a trainer, make sure he or she is experienced and that you feel comfortable in his or her presence. I realize that not everyone can hire a personal trainer due to financial situations and family needs, so that is why I have tried to make this book basic, practical, and functional.

Setting Up a Training Routine

The first question to ask yourself is how much time you can dedicate during the week for the gym. This, along with your goals, should determine how you're going to set up your training routine. For example, someone who can spare 30 minutes two or three days per week to train with weights will have a very different routine than someone who can go to the gym five or six days per week for an hour each day.

Another scenario is someone whose goal is general conditioning as opposed to someone who wants to add serious muscle while also becoming leaner—basicially someone who is looking to compete.

To give you some examples of routines to follow, I have developed four sample programs for various goals and needs. They will help you set up your own training routine based on the time and effort you can devote to training, along with your personal goals.

rotating between different body parts, you should not need a long rest period. In fact, as you become accustomed to this type of training, you should be able to go from one exercise to the next without resting. If you are at that stage, you will pause just long enough to set up your next exercise station.

This program is designed to be time-efficient, so it's important to just get it done. Wearing a watch and giving yourself a time frame to complete the workout will help to get the job done. Be disciplined!

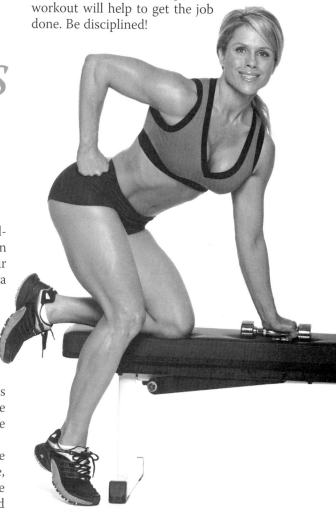

Sample Programs

Sample Training Program One:
Train Three Days per Week for General Conditioning

Each time in the gym you'll do a total-body circuit-training workout. You'll burn fat, shape your muscles, increase your energy, and feel better about yourself. In a circuit-style workout, you go from one exercise to another without resting in between, doing one set per exercise. For example, you may do one set of bicep curls, then a set of squats, then a set of flyes for chest. One total circuit (one set per exercise) is good; two circuits (one set per exercise, repeat circuit) are better; three (one set per exercise, done three times) is best.

If you are a beginner, rest no more than 30 seconds between each exercise, unless you feel very tired or winded. Since you're only doing one set per exercise and

Sample Training Program One
Three-Day Program

Body part	Exercise
Shoulders	Dumbbell press
Chest	Incline dumbbell press
Biceps	Seated alternating dumbbell curl
Triceps	Triceps bench dip
Back	Dumbbell bench row
Legs	Lunge
Abs	Basic ball crunch

Frequency

Three days per week
Monday/Wednesday/Friday or Tuesday/Thursday/Saturday

Exercise Selection

Pick one exercise per body part. (See sample above.) Select exercises from Exercise Descriptions, in the following section. If you do a second or third round, you may want to pick different exercises.

Sets

For each circuit, perform one set of each exercise. Repeat the circuit two or three times total, depending on the time you have that day and your conditioning level.

Reps

Do 15-20 reps per exercise. Add weight when you can do more than 20. It should not be so difficult that you can't do the last reps by yourself, but it should feel challenging enough that you're ready to quit at 20.

Rest

No more than 30 seconds between exercises

Cardio component

If you have the time, and these are the only three days you can get to the gym, do 15 minutes of cardio before your circuit and 15 minutes after your circuit. If you have a little bit more time, do 20 minutes before and 20 after. Do high-intensity cardio intervals so you get the most "bang for your buck"! (See explanation in the Cardiovascular Exercise section.)

Sample Training Program Two:
Train Four Days per Week for General Conditioning

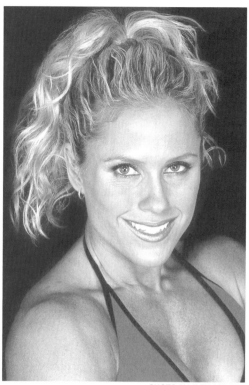

PHOTO BY ALEX ARDENTI

This is still a circuit-training workout, but your body parts are split between two days. The first circuit day focuses on arms (biceps and triceps) and legs. The second day you work your chest, shoulders and back.

Since your goals for circuit training are to burn fat while improving your conditioning, limit the amount of time you rest in between sets. Rest just long enough to set up your next workout station—usually less than 30 seconds between each exercise.

Adding a couple abdominal exercises into the mix one or two days a week should suffice for ab training. I prefer to superset my ab training into my upper-body circuits. I do not feel you need a separate workout just for abs unless you are an aspiring bodybuilder with weak abs. Keep in mind that abs get worked with almost all of your other workouts, so there is no need to overtrain them.

The 10 Most Important Minutes of Your Workout

Warming up is very important for both body and mind. You will find you're able to function in the gym more efficiently if you start your workout properly. You may have been sitting at a desk all day, so your body needs to acclimate to the next phase of activity. You'll increase the blood flow to your muscles and get your body heated up a bit so that you reduce your risk of pulling or tearing anything. You'll get your ligaments and tendons in gear so that your muscles can function properly.

Ten minutes is all you need to get a great warm up. It's a good amount of time to get your blood flowing and let the day's stress leave your mind so you can concentrate on your workout. I typically get on a treadmill and walk briskly for 10 minutes. You can start slowly, but work your way up to medium-intensity cardio, so your heart and lungs know it's time to exercise. I'll usually set the treadmill at about 3.5 mph with a five percent incline. That's medium intensity for me, but your chosen level may be higher or lower.

Planning your workout and visualizing the movements to come will help you get into your workout mode. I realize the time spent warming up is sometimes hard to come by, but I guarantee you will see better results both physically and mentally if you do not skip it—even five minutes will be better than none!

Sample Training Program Two

Four-Day Program

Frequency	Exercise
Monday	Arms/legs/abs
Tuesday	Chest/shoulders/back
Wednesday	Off
Thursday	Arms/legs/abs
Friday	Chest/shoulders/back
Saturday	Off
Sunday	Optional cardio day—perform more intense cardio where you're really focusing, doing intervals, a class, track work, intense hiking, or running on a slight incline.

Exercise Selection

Pick two exercises per body part. Select exercises from Exercise Descriptions, in the following section. If you do a second or third round, you may want to pick different exercises.

Sets

For each circuit, perform one set of each exercise. Repeat the circuit two or three times total, depending on the time you have that day.

Reps

Do 15-20 per exercise. Add weight when you can do more than 20. It should not be so difficult that you can't do the last reps by yourself, but it should feel challenging enough that you're ready to quit at 20.

Rest

No more than 30 seconds between exercises

Cardio Component

If time allows, include cardio before, after, or even in the middle of your circuit on your training days. Otherwise, save it for another day. I am a firm believer in doing cardio for fat loss and conditioning, so if you can include it, your results will be speedier. It doesn't have to be a long duration, but just something—even 15 minutes. Mix up your cardio, working at a lower intensity on some days, and a higher intensity on other days. Your energy level might dictate the amount and intensity of cardio you perform on a given day.

Sample Training Program Three:
Train Five Days a Week for Muscle Definition and Conditioning

This program is good for the woman who would like to build muscle definition throughout her entire body. This program is a three-day training split. Focus on chest, shoulders, and triceps the first day, doing two exercises for chest, three exercises for shoulders and two for triceps. The second day is back (three to four exercises), biceps (two exercises) and abs (two to three exercises). The third day is leg day (four exercises). The fourth day is a rest day, then return to the start of the three-day split.

Sample Training Program Three

Five-Day Program

Frequency	Exercise
Monday	Chest/shoulders/triceps
Tuesday	Back/biceps/abs
Wednesday	Legs
Thursday	Off or do cardio
Friday	Chest/shoulders/triceps
Saturday	Back/biceps/abs
Sunday	Off

Start with legs the following Monday. Tuesday is chest/shoulders/triceps, Wednesday is back/biceps/abs, and so forth. Writing down your schedule will definitely help you keep track of this type of regimen.

Exercise Selection	Pick from Exercise Descriptions (starting on page 26)
Chest	Two exercises
Shoulders	Three exercises
Triceps	Two exercises
Back	Three to four exercises
Biceps	Two exercises
Abs	Two to three exercises
Legs	Four exercises

Sets

Perform three to four sets per exercise, resting one minute in between sets.

Reps

Do 10-15—perform 15 reps for the first set, 12 for the second, and 10 for the third and optional fourth set.

Rest

One minute between sets

Cardio Component

I recommend doing some cardio for conditioning and to control body fat. Interval cardio sessions after weight training are best for optimal performance and results. Do not do your cardio before weights if you are trying to build muscle. Keep in mind that heavier training requires more attention and energy, so make sure you don't exhaust your fuel by doing your cardio first.

Sample Training
Program Four:
Four-Day Training Split for Muscle Development and Definition

This one is a little bit tricky, ladies; so read carefully! This is a typical four-day training split for someone dedicated to going to the gym and looking to build a considerable amount of muscle definition (possibly a fitness competitor). You'll lift heavier weights in this program and spend more time on each separate area of the body. Since you spend more time on individual body parts, you'll actually be training fewer body parts per day. The body is divided into four sections, as you'll see in the chart. In a given week you'll do the four-day split and then start again—meaning you'll actually be at the gym five days per week for this program. It's a four-day split, but you are at the gym five days per week—confusing, I know, but you'll get used to it in no time.

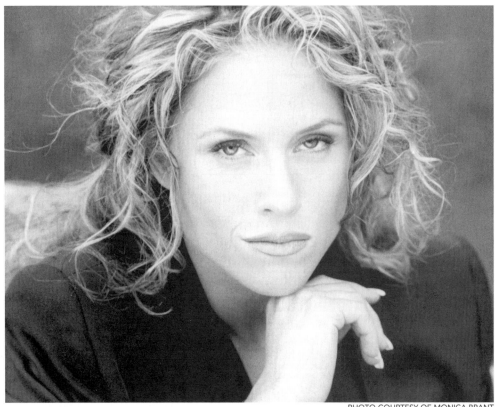

PHOTO COURTESY OF MONICA BRANT

Sample Training Program Four

Five-Day Program

Frequency	Exercise
Monday	Chest/arms/abs
Tuesday	Legs
Wednesday	Off
Thursday	Shoulders/abs
Friday	Back
Saturday	Off
Sunday	Chest/arms

As in sample program number three, you will again rotate the schedule depending on what day it is and what you trained last. Writing down the days/workouts will help you remember. In the above example, the next Monday will be legs, Tuesday will be an off day and Wednesday will be shoulders.

Exercise Selection	Pick from Exercise Description
Chest	Two exercises
Triceps	Three exercises
Biceps	Two exercises
Abs	Two to three exercises
Legs	Four exercises
Shoulders	Four exercises
Back	Four exercises

Sets

Perform four sets per exercise.

Reps

Do 12 for the first set, 12 for the second set, 10 for the third set, and eight for the fourth set.

Rest

No more than 60-90 seconds between sets

Cardio Component

See Sample Training Program Three. For best results in building muscle, do your cardio after weight training or on other (non-weight training) days.

Learning the Terms

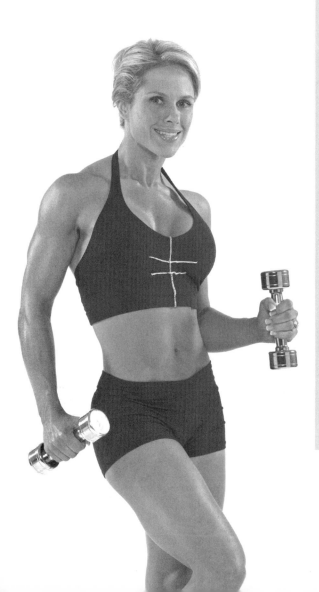

I want to clarify what I mean when I use certain terms such as supersets, giant sets and circuits. You can use these important training techniques to manipulate your workouts and hopefully get quicker results, bringing you one step closer to achieving your goals.

Supersets: With this technique, go from one exercise to the next without resting. The exercises should target opposing muscle groups. For example, start with one set of triceps kickbacks and immediately switch to a wide-grip biceps curl. Since you're working opposing muscle groups, the biceps will be ready to go even though you just worked your triceps. There should generally be no resting in between the exercises, but do rest for a brief 30-60 seconds before performing the first exercise of the two again.

Giant Sets: With this challenging technique, perform three to four exercises in a row (one set for each exercise). Do not rest in between exercises, but do rest after the last exercise since you'll definitely need a break before beginning your second "giant set." A killer example of a giant set is a leg press, followed by a leg curl, followed immediately with a leg extension. You'll deserve that rest for 60 seconds after the leg extension! Since giant sets are such an intense training technique, try mixing up your workouts and doing giant sets periodically for a change of pace.

Circuits: Circuit training is similar to doing a giant set. You basically perform one exercise after another with no rest in between. My "rest" will often be going to the cardio machine for 10 minutes in between sets, as I discuss later in my training section. I will do circuit training for lower-body workouts, upper-body workouts and, at times, upper and lower mixed for variety. Circuits are one of the best ways to burn fat and condition your body.

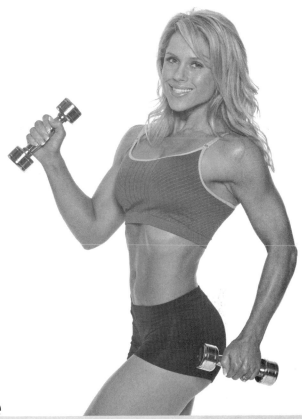

Mental Muscle

Many people zone out when they train, but I like to concentrate on what I'm doing, setting aside all other thoughts from the day. This guarantees that I will not slack off during my workout and help me make the most of the time I am spending in the gym. Keep in mind that in my line of work, my training sessions directly relate to my income!

If I allow myself to slip and become lethargic, my physique will start to show my poor work ethic. This is one of the reasons I do not listen to music while I train. The other reason is simply that I don't want to have to think about extra things before heading to the gym. It is enough to make sure I have my straps, heart-rate monitor, towel, water and any supplements that I will need after training. This is my time to be in the gym, focusing on what is needed for that hour or so and not thinking of anything else.

Wearing a watch will help keep you aware of your rest times and overall schedule. When you enter the gym, make a mental note of what time you expect to be finished and when you will need to eat afterwards. (We will get to the nutrition "dos and don'ts" later on, but keep in mind that you do not want to wait more than 60 minutes after your workout to eat some good carbohydrates and protein.)

I realize no one has time to waste, so make the most of every second. If someone wants to chat while you are training, be firm yet friendly and tell them you are on a tight schedule with your training and that you will have to catch up with them another time. Remember that some people come to the gym solely to have some company. Do not feel badly—just be honest. Maybe it will encourage them to be more diligent in their workouts! Or, if it is someone you enjoy, ask them to join you in your workout.

People sometimes ask me, how long is too long to be in the gym? I think an hour to an hour and a half is plenty. Without the unnecessary chitchat you should be able to get everything done in that amount of time and be on your way.

Exercise
Descriptions

Shoulders (also called Deltoids)
Four exercises total

Dumbbell Press

Sit on a bench (preferably a bench with a back support) holding two dumbbells at the sides of your upper chest (near level with your shoulders), with your palms facing forward. The bench should be set to a 90-degree angle. Press both arms straight overhead. Be careful to keep your shoulders stationary—they shouldn't hunch up. Proper upper-body stretching will increase your ability to do this particular exercise effectively. Bring your arms back down so that the weights are about even with the tops of your shoulders. Repeat, keeping the movement fluid throughout.

Pace: Three seconds up, three seconds down.

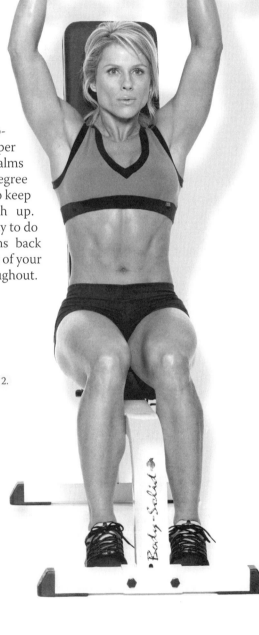

2.

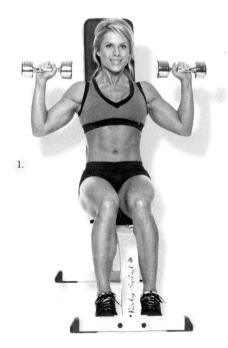

1.

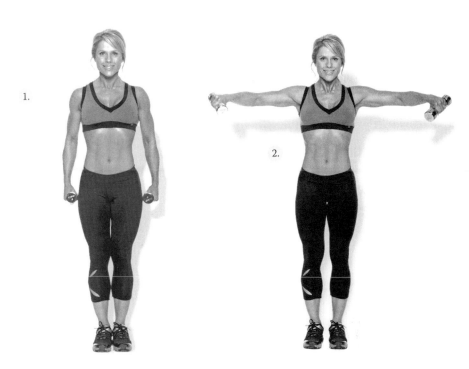

Side Lateral Raise

Stand with feet together, holding a pair of dumbbells in your hands. Your palms should face your outer thighs. Bring your arms up in an arc, lifting from your elbows rather than your hands. If you look at the dumbbell, your hands should be shifted slightly toward the back, rather than the front of the weight. Pretend there is a string lifting your elbows up. Maintain a very slight bend in your arm, rather than locking it straight out. Go up until your arms are parallel to the ground, making sure your hands do not rise above shoulder level. Bring your arms down and repeat. The movement should be fluid, smooth and controlled.

Pace: Three seconds up, three seconds down.

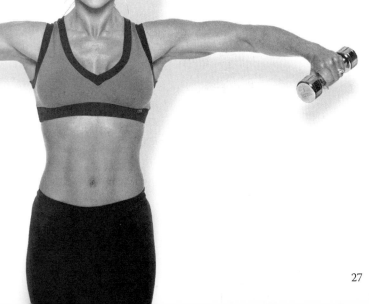

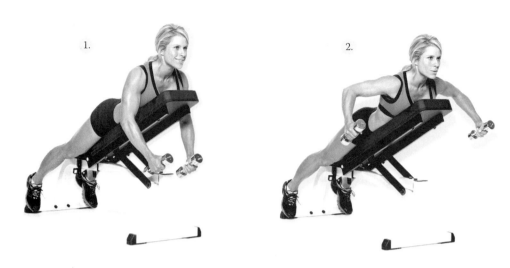

1.   2.

Bench Rear Delt Flye

Set a bench to a 45-degree angle, and sit with your chest resting against the pad. Your chin should be just over the top of the seat. Foot position depends upon how tall you are—I'm on the shorter side, so I rest my toes on the bottom leg of the bench so I don't slip. Start with your palms facing in, your arms hanging down with a slight bend in your elbows. The weights should hang straight down from your shoulders. Keeping your elbows bent, lift your arms until they are about parallel with the floor. If you feel the movement in your back, you're doing more of a rowing motion than a flye. Done properly, you will feel the movement in the rear section of your shoulders. Going slow, focusing on the movement, and watching in the mirror will ensure you maintain proper form.

Pace: Three seconds up, three seconds down.

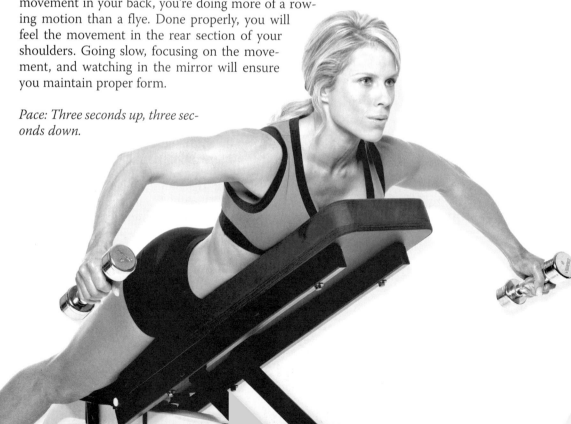

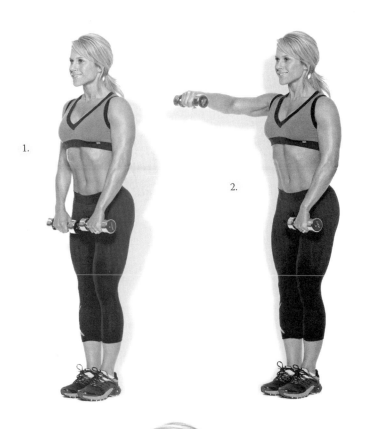

1.

2.

♡ *Shoulder*
  Training Notes

- Don't be afraid to allow your neck to loosen up in between reps if you feel it tightening. Just briefly stop at the bottom of the movement and allow your neck to relax.

- Take deep breaths, inhaling through your nose and exhaling through your mouth. These deep breaths will help you deliver the maximum amount of oxygen to your muscles and help you stay as relaxed as possible. Inhale on the way up with the movements and exhale on the way down.

Front Lateral Raise

Stand with feet together, holding a pair of dumbbells with palms facing the front of your thighs. Keep your left arm at your side and raise your right arm until it is parallel with the floor. Don't lock out your elbow; instead keep it very slightly bent. Slowly lower your right arm in a controlled manner. Repeat with your left side and continue to alternate arms for the desired number of repetitions. Come up only until your arm is parallel to the floor, no higher.

Pace: Three seconds up, three seconds down.

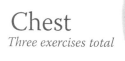

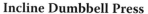

Chest
Three exercises total

Incline Dumbbell Press

Sit on an incline bench set to about 45 degrees. Hold a pair of dumbbells at your sides. Bend your elbows and raise the weights to about mid-chest level, with palms facing outward. Press up in a small arc, bringing the weights together at the top and squeezing your chest muscles as you press. In a smooth and controlled manner, retrace your arc as you return the weights to chest level.

To help with proper form (and to be lady-like), I prefer to keep my knees together and hold my abs tight, pushing my lower back down. Don't arch your lower back! As you return to the lower position, the weights should almost reach shoulder level—don't drop lower than that, or you'll strain your shoulders.

Pace: Three seconds up, three seconds down.

Going to the Gym vs. Training at Home?

At this time in my life, I do not have any home equipment; therefore if I want to train, I must head to the gym. However, if I had the equipment, I might prefer to get some of my workouts in at home—that is if I could avoid getting distracted by the computer, phone calls, laundry and other household duties, and procrastination (putting off working out until too late and by then I am too tired).

If you have the equipment at home and are capable of getting your workouts done, I applaud your discipline! For me, going to the gym provides me with motivation to stop all other activities and focus my attention strictly on my workout. And it reminds me that I am not alone in my quest for a better physique!

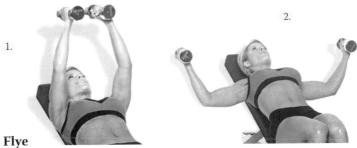

1.

2.

Incline Dumbbell Flye

Sit on an incline bench set to about 45 degrees. Hold a pair of dumbbells at your sides. To start, press the weights straight up over your chest, with elbows slightly bent and palms facing each other. In a smooth and controlled manner, lower the weights to the sides in an arc, keeping your elbows slightly bent. Stop when your elbows are parallel to the floor, or even before parallel if that is more comfortable for your range of motion. Again, bring the weights together at the top, squeezing your chest at the top of the movement. (There's no need to clank the weights together at the top.) As you lower the weight each time, don't drop back too far, or you'll strain your shoulder joints. Also, do not let the weights go lower than the crowns of your shoulders.

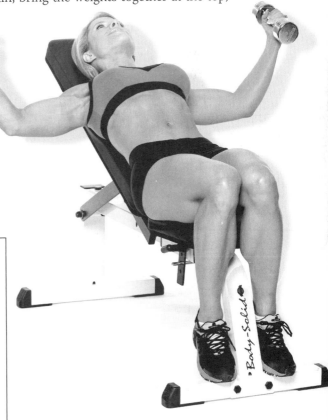

Pace: Three seconds up, three seconds down.

♥ Chest Training Notes

• I prefer to do chest training on an incline, and I advise that most women do the same. I don't feel it is necessary to do flat bench work—unless of course you are an aspiring bodybuilder.

• Don't forget your breathing, inhaling on the way up and exhaling on the way down.

• Keep in mind that you may feel some tricep soreness after an intense chest routine. This is normal, since triceps are the secondary muscle worked on many chest exercises—especially if you incorporate pushups!

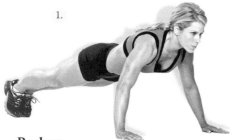

1.

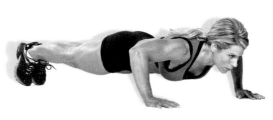

2.

Pushup

If you are a beginner or cannot do pushups on your toes, begin on your knees and progress to your toes as you get stronger. To begin a regular pushup, hold your body straight with your toes and hands touching the ground. Hands should be just outside of shoulder-width apart. Lower your body toward the ground and then lift back up. You should go down until your upper arms are parallel with the floor—don't go lower, or you will place unnecessary strain on your shoulder joints. Keep your neck and spine in alignment, and don't let the middle of your body sag. Your abs should remain tight. If you cannot maintain a straight-body position, drop to your knees and finish the desired amount of repetitions.

Pace: Two seconds up, two seconds down.

Alternate Positioning

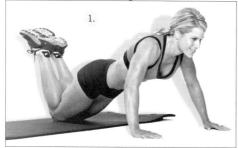

1.

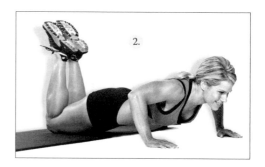

2.

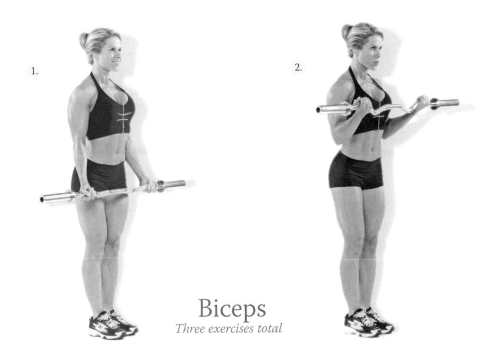

Biceps

Three exercises total

EZ-Curl with Wide Grip

Stand with feet about hip-width apart and your knees slightly bent. Hold an EZ-Curl bar at thigh level with a wide underhand grip. Raise the bar up to chest height, keeping your upper arms stationary. Don't bring your arms up fully, or you'll lose the contraction in your biceps. Also, when you return the bar to thigh level, keep a slight bend in your elbows so you don't lose the contraction at the bottom. Focus on squeezing your biceps as you raise the weight and keep your abs tight throughout the movement.

Pace: Three seconds up, three seconds down.

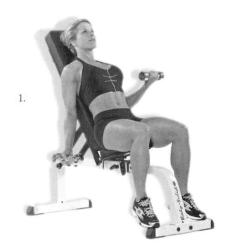

1.

Seated Alternating Dumbbell Curl

Sit on a bench set to about a 75-degree angle, holding a pair of dumbbells at your sides. Your palms should face forward. Alternate each arm, beginning with your right. Raise the dumbbell to slightly below mid-chest level, keeping your palms in the same face-up position (don't twist your wrists). Continue alternating each arm for the desired amount of repetitions.

Pace: Three seconds up, three seconds down.

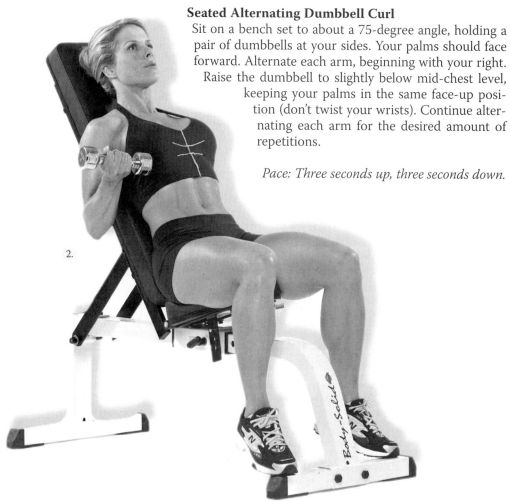

2.

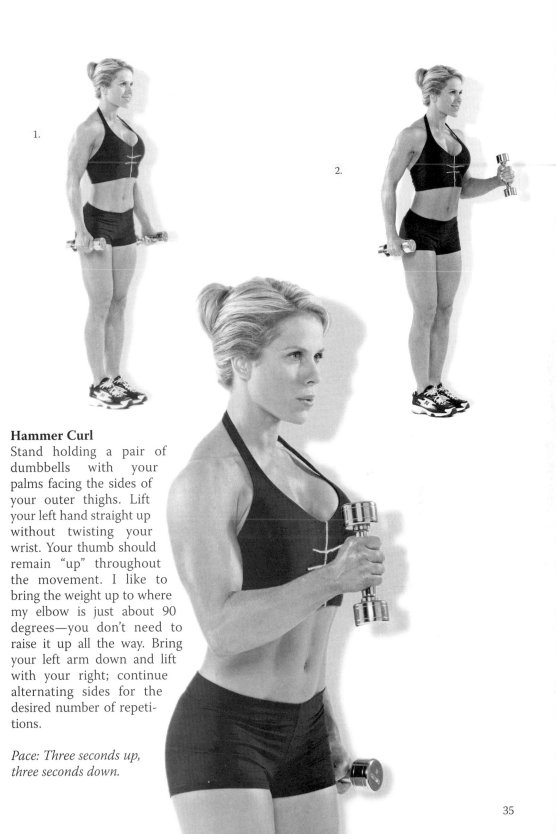

1.

2.

Hammer Curl

Stand holding a pair of dumbbells with your palms facing the sides of your outer thighs. Lift your left hand straight up without twisting your wrist. Your thumb should remain "up" throughout the movement. I like to bring the weight up to where my elbow is just about 90 degrees—you don't need to raise it up all the way. Bring your left arm down and lift with your right; continue alternating sides for the desired number of repetitions.

Pace: Three seconds up, three seconds down.

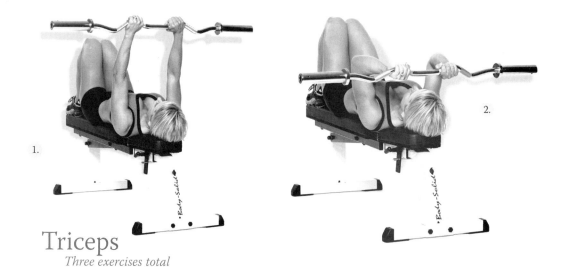

1.

2.

Triceps
Three exercises total

Overhead EZ-Curl Press

Lie on a bench and hold an EZ-Curl bar with straight arms over your head. I prefer to bend my knees and put my feet on the bench, because it helps my back remain flat, not arched. If you're taller or it's more comfortable for you, keep your feet on the ground. Bring the weight down so that the tops of your hands are about six inches from your forehead. At this point your forearms should be parallel to the floor—you don't want to drop lower than that, or you'll start straining your tendons. Your upper arms should remain stationary throughout the movement. Your wrists should not bend. To return, press your lower arms back up so that your arms are again overhead but your elbows are slightly bent. Don't "lock out" your arms by bringing them to full extension. Think about keeping your elbows together; as you fatigue, they tend to wander out.

Pace: Three seconds up, three seconds down.

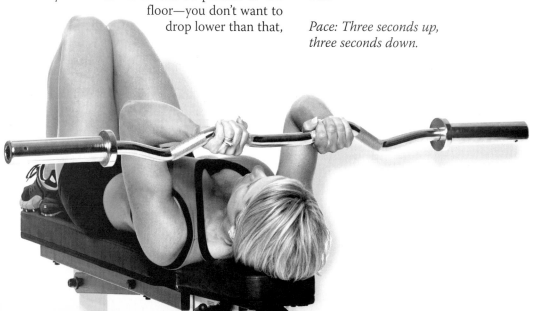

Dumbbell Kickback

Rest your left knee on a bench and keep your right foot straight on the ground. Hold the edge of the bench with your left hand, and grasp a dumbbell with your right hand. (I have weak wrists, so I don't put my hand flat on the bench for support. Instead I hold the edge of the bench to put my wrist in a better position.) Keep your abs tight and chest slightly up. Focus your eyes forward, not down. Again, the mirror will help ensure that your form is correct throughout the movement. Start with your right elbow bent at 90 degrees and close to your body.

1.

Extend it back fully so that your entire right arm is straight behind you. Then, bring your arm back to the 90-degree angle in a slow and controlled manner. Don't let the weight drop or swing back. This is a very short range of motion—it starts at the hip and goes back only about six to eight inches. Do all the repetitions on your right side, then switch to your left side.

Pace: Three seconds up, three seconds down.

2.

♡ *Triceps Training Notes*

- Be sure to really concentrate on flexing your triceps at the top of each movement. You should feel a good squeeze each time!

- Again, your breathing is important, inhaling on the up and exhaling on the down.

Triceps Bench Dip

Sit on a bench with your hands just outside of your hips and palms on the bench. Place your feet on the floor, then lower your body toward the floor by bending your arms and keeping your lower body still. I lower myself until my upper arms are about parallel to the floor, then push back up. I then squeeze my triceps at the top of the movement. You may not be able to go so far down right away, so just go to a point that is comfortable for you, where you're able to maintain control. Also, the more your knees are bent, the easier the movement is.

Keep your back close to the bench, so you target your triceps rather than your shoulders. As with most triceps exercises, keep your elbows close to

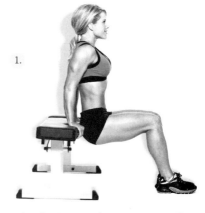

1.

your body. Remember, triceps will wander outward as they fatigue, allowing another muscle group to try and take over! To make the movement more difficult: place your feet farther out in front of you; place a stability ball under your feet; or place your feet on another bench in front of you, with a weight on your lap for added resistance.

Pace: Three seconds up, three seconds down.

2.

Back
Four exercises total

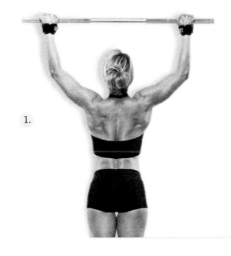

1.

Pull-up

Pull-ups are definitely one of the hardest exercises for me, yet they are one of my favorites, too! My entire back has unquestionably become stronger since I incorporated pull-ups into my back training routine.

Fortunately, pull-ups can be done in a variety of methods. Of course, doing them on your own with a simple chin bar should be the ultimate goal. For those of you who have never done pull-ups before, I suggest locating the assisted pull-up machine (the machine lifts part of your body weight for you) in your gym to get acquainted with this challenging exercise. Once you have mastered the assisted pull-up machine (sometimes called the Gravitron), find an experienced "spotter" to help you use the simple chin bar, as this will be more difficult than the assisted pull-up machine.

Now listen up, ladies…Please keep in mind that women are typically stronger in their lower bodies and carry more weight in their legs, which makes pull-ups harder. But don't let that be an excuse to NOT do pull-ups! As long as you can physically do this exercise, I urge you to add them to your routine.

I like to perform pull-ups with a wide overhand grip (just outside of shoulder width) and use a training product called Versa Gripps to help me get a better grip on the bar. These two things force my back to work, not my hands and forearms. (Read more details in Back Training Notes.)

To do a pull-up, stand on a platform or flat bench, grip the bar, and pull your chest upward using your back muscles. Try to get your chin close to the bar.

Just for your information…I can only do seven or eight—maybe 10 on a good day—on my first set. I do four to five sets of pull-ups, usually with a spotter.

Pace: Three seconds up,
three seconds down (if you can).

2.

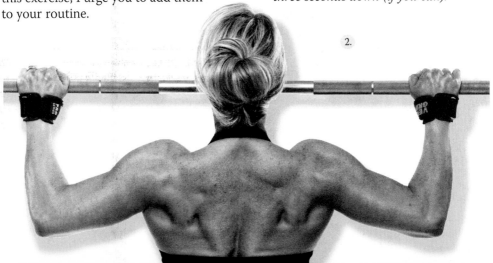

One-Arm Dumbbell Row

Place your left knee and hand on a bench. While your right foot stays on the floor, grasp a dumbbell with your right hand. Your right (working) arm should hang down close to your body. I like to keep my working arm close to my side throughout the movement. Using your back muscles, pull your right elbow up until your arm is bent at about a 90-degree angle. The motion is like sawing wood—from your armpit to your hip and back down again. At the top of the movement I like to visualize trying to bring my elbow over my back—it's a slight extra squeeze that's very effective. Do the desired number of repetitions with your right side, and then switch to your left, making sure to do an even amount on both sides. Keep your eyes focused in front of you and your back straight during each repetition.

Pace: Three seconds up, three seconds down.

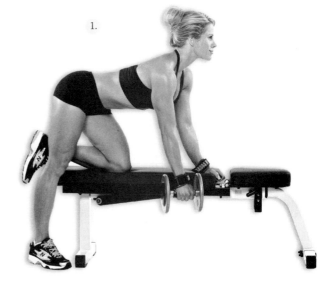

1.

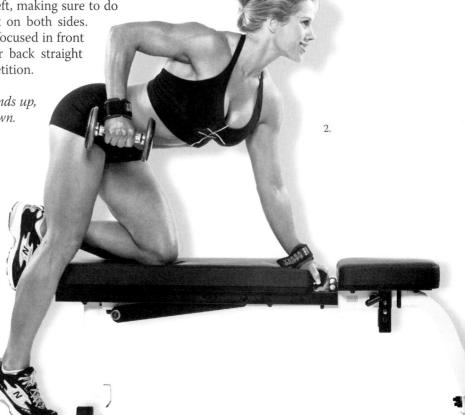

2.

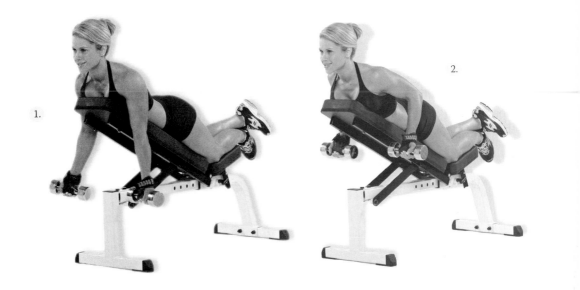

1.

2.

Dumbbell Bench Row

Set a bench to a 45-degree angle and sit with your belly resting against the back-rest and your knees resting on the seat. (If you're tall, you can sit on the seat with your feet on the floor and your belly resting against the backrest.) Use a reverse (underhand) grip as you hold two dumb-bells. Begin with your arms hanging down and then pull your arms behind you, using your back muscles as you pull. Go until your arm reaches about a 90-degree angle. Keep your arms close to the sides of your body throughout the movement and your eyes focused in front of you.

Pace: Three seconds up, three seconds down.

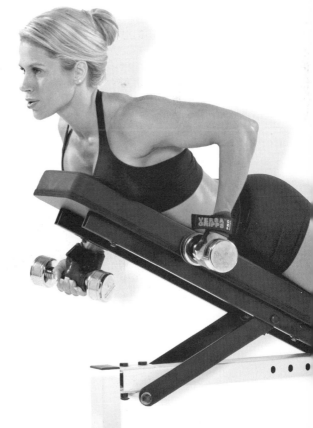

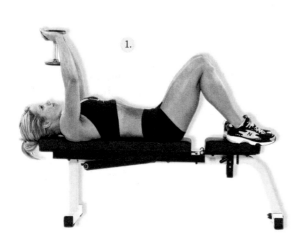

1.

Dumbbell Pullover

Lie on a flat bench with your knees bent and your feet on the edge of the bench so that
your low back is flat. Place the *palms* of your hands against the inside face of the dumbbell. Start with your arms straight up overhead, then bring your arms backward and
down, until they are nearly parallel with the floor. Your back should stay flat on the
bench, with your abs held tight. If your back is arching, you're either going back too far
or the weight is too heavy to handle properly. Keep a slight bend in your elbows throughout the movement, but keep your arms rigid. If you feel this in your triceps, you're probably bending your elbows too much. Since this is a stretching exercise, start with a light
weight until you build your strength and perfect your form.

Pace: Three seconds up, three seconds down.

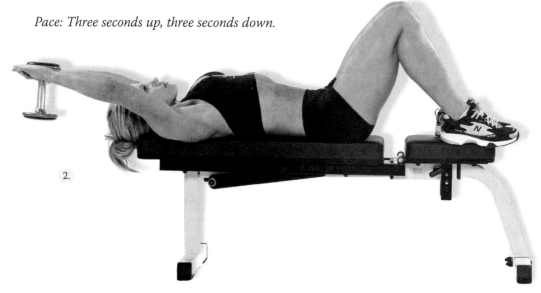

2.

Legs and Glutes
Four exercises total

1.

Lunge

Another of my favorite exercises is the lunge and, when I exercise, I perform one of the many variations with every leg routine.

Some examples of beginner lunges are:

- Stationary—one leg at a time
- Stationary—alternating legs
- Walking
- On a Smith machine, to help with your balance and form

Examples of more advanced lunges include:

- Walking with a kick to the rear for a great glute workout
- Walking with a high knee lift to the front for some hip flexor work
- Walking and combining both the rear kick and the front knee lift
- Lunge with your front foot up on a small box/platform
- Lunge with your rear toe up on a bench or box/platform

Unless you are using the Smith machine, holding dumbbells at your side or placing a small weight bar on your shoulders will increase the workload. If you want more of a cardio effect, use very light dumbbells and do reps of 20-30 per leg. Using dumbbells will also help with your balance if you are new to lunges.

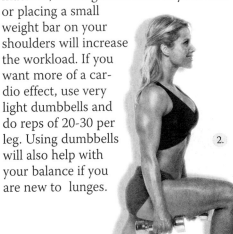

2.

To perform a basic lunge, first stand with your feet together. Take a big step forward with your right foot and plant it on the ground in front of you. Your torso should be balanced between your front and back legs, not leaning forward or back. I find most people make the mistake of keeping their feet too close, which adds extra strain on their knees. Make sure to step forward with an extra long stride and then bring your front foot back a bit if necessary before starting.

Rise up on your ball of your back foot and lower your body down, keeping your body on one plane. Remember: Don't lean forward or back—you will tend to do this as you fatigue! Stop when your front knee reaches a 90-degree angle. Form is important! Do not allow your back knee to touch (or bang!) the floor, and do not allow your front knee to extend over your front toe. Push through the heel of your forward foot the whole time, and squeeze your glutes as you come back up. It's almost an automatic squeeze if you're pushing through that front heel. Throughout the movement, keep your abs tight, eyes looking forward, chin up, and shoulders back. I think it's easier to do all the reps on one foot and stay in a stationary position, rather than repositioning yourself each time. I realize this is a lot to remember, but you can do it! Your glutes, hams, quads and calves will thank you, as will your honey!

Pace: Two seconds up, two seconds down.

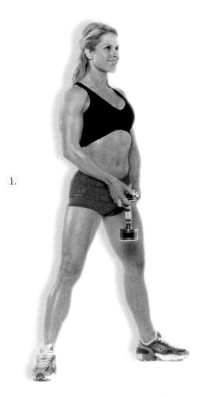

1.

2.

Dumbbell Plié Squat

Stand straight up, holding one dumbbell with two hands in front of your thighs. You should hold the weight by interlacing your fingers in a palms-up position at the top of the weight. Take a plié position with your feet wider than shoulder-width apart and your toes slightly pointed out. Lower your body down, keeping your rear end tucked underneath you—don't let it travel out. Keeping your back straight and abs tight, go down as far as is comfortable for you, stopping just before your upper thighs are parallel with the ground. Make sure your knees don't travel inward as you fatigue. When I'm going down I concentrate on my outer thighs; when I'm coming up I squeeze my glutes and inner thighs.

Pace: Three seconds up, three seconds down.

Stiff-Legged Deadlift

Stand with your feet together, holding a barbell or pair of dumbbells in front of you. If you use a barbell you can either use an underhand grip for both hands or an alternating grip (one palm facing my body, one facing away); if I do them with dumbbells, my palms face my thighs.

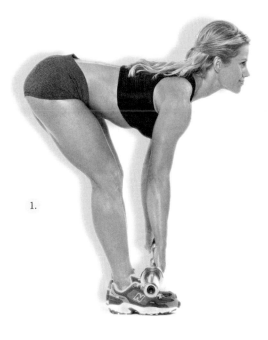

1.

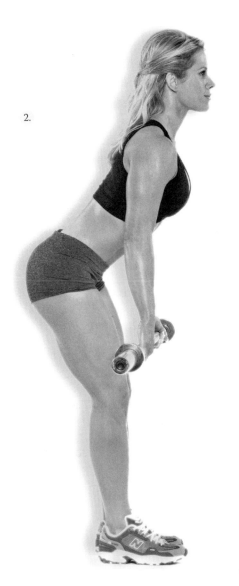

2.

Definitely do these with a light weight in the beginning, because you don't want to overstretch your hamstrings. Lower the weight down to below knee level (you don't need to drop it to your feet), keeping your chest lifted, shoulders back, abs tight, eyes level and back straight. Depending on your flexibility, go from below the knee to about knee or mid-thigh level, but definitely stop by mid-thigh level. You don't want to stand all the way up. Keep the weight close to your body and maintain a slight bend in your knees. Squeeze your hamstrings and glutes as you come up each time.

Pace: Three seconds up, three seconds down.

1.

Step-Up

Stand in front of a low, sturdy bench, or stack a few steps together (as shown). Don't use a bench with a lot of padding, because it's harder to balance your foot on the bench. Place your right foot on the step, and bend your left knee slightly. Press up forcefully through your right foot as you raise your body up. Make sure your full foot is on the bench, not just the ball of your foot.

I usually do all the reps on one leg before switching legs. In that case, my working foot will remain on the bench the whole time as I lift and lower my body. When you're stepping up, push through your heel and squeeze your glutes. When you lower yourself, control the descent and don't allow your body to just fall back to the floor. Try not to push off with the foot that's on the floor too much. The slower you go, the harder the exercise becomes.

Regarding knee position, your knee should never go past 90 degrees. The range of motion is the same for beginners and advanced trainers. It's the height of the step that determines the difficulty.

If you do all of the reps on one side before switching legs, alternate so you don't always start with the same leg. The leg that goes first is usually going to be working harder. Make sure you do the same amount of reps on each leg. Beginners may want to alternate legs for each rep. (If you alternate legs, you'll return to a legs-together position between each rep.)

To make this exercise more difficult, hold a pair of dumbbells in your hands. Start with light weights and gradually increase as you're comfortable with the movement. For a real challenge, incorporate a backward kick into each rep. To do this, as you come up and your working leg is on the bench, kick the *opposite* leg backward. For this variation, you should definitely hold dumbbells, because they help give you better balance between the front and back of your body.

This is not like step class, in which you use momentum and swing your arms. It's a slow, controlled movement.

Pace: The pace for this exercise is faster than the others. If the bench is lower, the pace will be shorter—maybe just a second up and a second down. The higher the bench, the longer it will take to go up and down. As you fatigue, just concentrate on the form and keeping your knees in alignment rather than maintaining a certain pace.

2.

❧ Legs
Training Notes

- I do mostly circuit training for legs, using very low weights and high reps. Sometimes I use no added weight at all and let my body weight be the only resistance. At times I'll go up to 50 reps per exercise. I have been training this way for many years now since I am not trying to gain any new muscle in my legs. I'm just focusing on conditioning and strengthening.

- For a sample indoor leg workout, I'll do 20-30 minutes on a stepmill or treadmill set to a high incline. I'll keep my heart rate at 60-75% of maximum, using my Polar heart-rate monitor for ease and accuracy. Then I'll do a leg circuit with four or five exercises for 25-30 reps each. Then it's another 10 minutes of cardio, another leg circuit, then back to cardio for 10 minutes. This type of workout will typically last an hour and a half and will drain me of all my energy!

- Keeping both legs evenly strengthened is important to me, so I do many one-legged exercises, such as lunges, leg press/sleds, leg extensions, and leg curls.

- If I am not doing a circuit routine, I will superset my leg exercises. For example, I might do a set of lunges and immediately do a set of squats.

- Lunges are one of the best overall leg conditioning exercises. They target your entire leg (and get your heart rate up). For more advanced moves, try walking lunges and walking lunges with a kick for an extra glute squeeze. All the basic elements are the same for a walking lunge, you're just moving forward. It's very important that your body remains in the same plane, straight up and straight down. As you fatigue, you'll automatically want to lean forward, so go slow to keep your body properly positioned. Take a long enough step so that you will not extend your knee past your toe. It does take practice to gain your balance and feel comfortable. Do not feel bad if walking lunges are hard for you to do. It will take some time to gain your balance and feel comfortable with this exercise. Once you master the walking lunge, you'll be lunging around the perimeter of the gym. I've even seen many people outside the gym, lunging around the parking lot since the gyms typically do not have enough open floor space. If your gym's aerobic room is empty, do your lunges there, as there will be ample space, and you will not worry about running into anyone.

- I typically do not train calves, mostly because of all the running I incorporate into my workouts. All the box jumping, sprinting, bleachers, and plyometric exercises keep them conditioned. If you want to target your calves with weights, just do standard calf raises. The calf-training machines in the gym are pretty self-explanatory. Keep in mind that calves seem to be a very genetic muscle group. You either have them or you don't! They can grow, but you need to be patient and consistent. When training calves, it's most important to do all three foot positions—heels out, heels in and feet straight. Do a full range of motion, going all the way up and all the way down.

- I thoroughly enjoy getting away from the gym as much as possible, and heading to the track is definitely one of my all-time favorite training pastimes! If slimmer body lines and conditioned, round glutes are one of your priorities, try sprinting. If you are like me, I can guarantee that is music to your ears! With every track workout I combine any of the following: plyometrics, stadium stairs/bleachers, sprinting, and foot drills. I realize not everyone has the beautiful Southern California weather to take advantage of, so I suggest that you locate an indoor track at a local college or find a nearby fitness facility that provides one when those outdoor temperatures are too cold to handle. Maybe you will find someone there who inspires you more than in the gym. For me, it has been a motivating factor to watch the Olympic athletes in training—they make it look so easy. If only it was!

1.

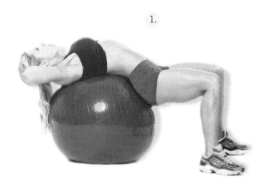

2.

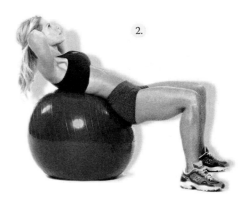

Abs
Four exercises total

3.

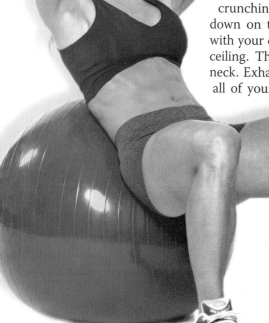

Basic Ball Crunch

Sit on an exercise ball and balance yourself by walking your feet out in front of you into a wide foot position. Place your hands behind your lower head and upper neck for support and lower yourself until your back is supported by the ball. Then, using your abs, lift your upper body, crunching down on your abs. Don't slide too far down on the ball. Keep your eyes focused upwards, with your chin up. I like to focus on one spot near the ceiling. This will help keep you from straining your neck. Exhale on the way up, making sure to blow out all of your air at the top to fully contract your abs. Inhale on the way down.

Pace: Three seconds up, three seconds down.

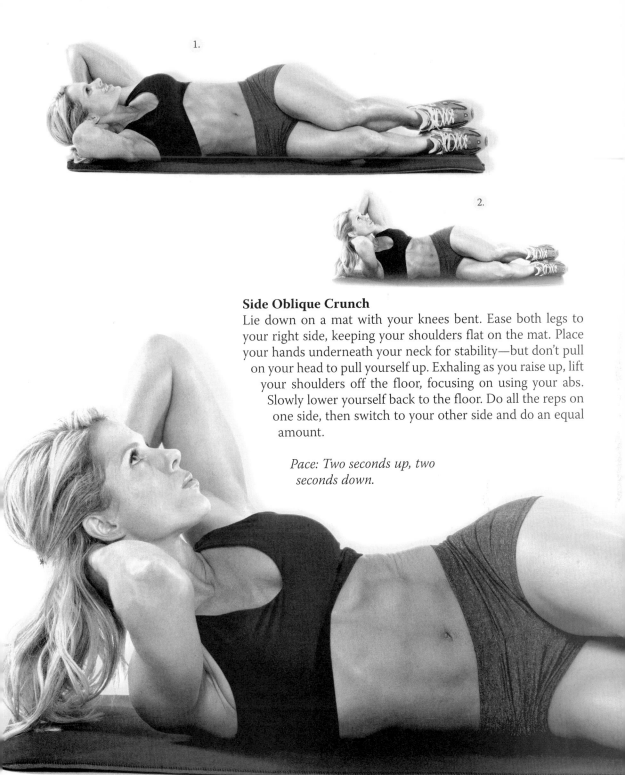

Side Oblique Crunch

Lie down on a mat with your knees bent. Ease both legs to your right side, keeping your shoulders flat on the mat. Place your hands underneath your neck for stability—but don't pull on your head to pull yourself up. Exhaling as you raise up, lift your shoulders off the floor, focusing on using your abs. Slowly lower yourself back to the floor. Do all the reps on one side, then switch to your other side and do an equal amount.

Pace: Two seconds up, two seconds down.

Alternating Straight Leg Raises

This is a scissors-like movement in which you alternate legs, bringing each leg up above the other. Lie on a flat bench or mat and cross your hands behind your neck. If you need some extra help with balance, try placing your hands beneath your hips. Bring each leg up in a slow, controlled movement, focusing on your lower abdominal region and keeping your low back flat on the bench or mat. Alternate the legs for an even number, rest, and repeat. This exercise does target the hip flexors as well as the abs, so be careful not to overexert them if you are just starting out. To make this exercise more difficult, raise both legs together!

Pace: Three seconds up, three seconds down.

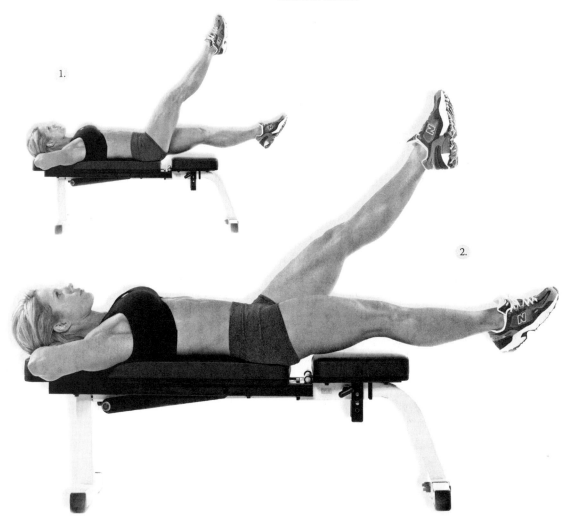

1.

2.

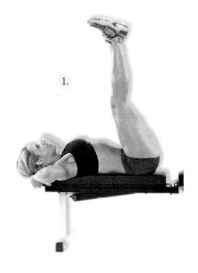

1.

Hip Thrust on Bench

Lie down on a bench and grasp the edges under your head. Bend at your hips so that your legs are in the air, knees slightly bent, with the soles of your feet pointing to the ceiling. Raise your hips four to six inches off the bench—just enough to feel your lower abdominal region squeezing. Do not try to go too high by using your hands as leverage.

Remember: Your feet should go straight up and down, not swinging forward and/or backward. For that extra squeeze, I exhale on the up movement, blowing out my entire breath before inhaling and coming back to the start position.

Pace: Two seconds up,
two seconds down.

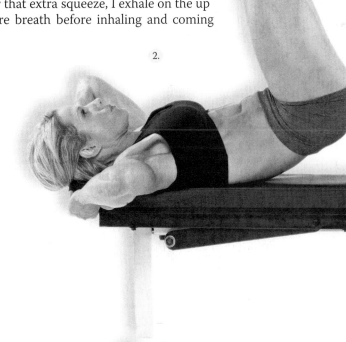

2.

❦ Ab Training Notes

• I prefer to do ab exercises with my hands behind my neck, because my neck starts hurting without that support. I just try to always be conscious of not pulling my neck—the hands are only there for stability.

• Don't forget to breathe correctly. Exhale on the "working" part of the exercise and inhale on the negative.

Cardiovascular Exercise

The many important benefits of cardiovascular exercise include strengthening your heart, losing body fat, gaining energy and relieving stress. Also known as aerobic exercise, cardio can be described as any activity that causes you to use large muscle groups in a continuous method. There are many activities that fit this description, so be sure to choose one (or more) that you enjoy and are capable of performing. Giving yourself a variety will ensure that you don't become bored and unenthusiastic.

How long should you do cardio?

It will definitely depend on your fitness level. For those of you who are beginners, start with 20 to 25 minutes, two to three times a week. After this feels good and you see improvements in your endurance, bump up the time to 30-40 minutes, three to four times weekly.

At that point you will be on your way to ultimate Cardio Queen status, making 60 minutes a feather in your cap! If you go for the complete hour, make sure to take in enough nutrients for your body. If not, you will risk losing that hard-earned muscle from being over-trained and undernourished. This is not the ideal setting for your body to recover and grow efficiently.

What is the best time of day to do cardio?

This is definitely a controversial topic. In my humble opinion, the best time is the time you can do it! I have yet to experience a specific time that yields better results than others for optimal fat loss. However, my preference is cardio in the morning after I have finished a whey protein shake made only with water. After consuming this shake, I wait 30 minutes and then go for a good run outside. The protein seems to refresh and refuel my body after "fasting" through the night—keeping me from feeling depleted, as I would on an empty stomach. My second favorite time for cardio is immediately following an intense weight training session.

What types of cardio should I choose?

In the gym, choose among the treadmill, elliptical machine, stair climber, bike, and aerobics classes. Out of the gym, there's fast walking, jogging, running, cycling, inline skating, hiking, and, of course, track work such as bleachers and sprinting.

What method of cardio is best?

The two basic categories of cardio exercise are the "Long and Slow" method and the "Interval" method.

Long and Slow: This slow and steady method is a more traditional way of training. It's genuine "aerobic" exercise, described in the dictionary as occurring only in the presence of oxygen, involving or improving oxygen consumption by the body. For "long and slow" cardio, you should maintain about the same heart rate and level of intensity for a given amount of time. For this type of cardio to be effective, stay in a range of 5 to 7, given a scale of 1 to 10 (10 being all-out maximum effort and 1 being "why bother, you might as well be snoozing").

Interval: With interval training you alternate periods of high intensity (anaerobic) and low intensity (aerobic) cardio. The dictionary describes "anaerobic" as occurring in the absence of free oxygen...during heavy exercise anaerobic respiration occurs.

The intervals can be as long or short as you desire or can handle, but generally you should warm up (there's that ol' warm up thing again!), then alternate between two minutes of high-intensity hard work (7-8 range) and two minutes of recovery (4-6 range).

If I'm doing sprints outside, I might sprint 70 to 85 meters (high intensity) and then jog back (lower intensity). If I am inside on the stepmill, I split up my time with intervals whenever I feel like it. I might do one intense interval every five minutes, or alternate every 30 seconds for 10 minutes straight.

Just about any combination of intervals will work and be effective. It's typically easy enough to figure out how to make the machines harder. Raising the incline or speed will definitely bring up your heart rate. Try upping the intensity and see how much you can handle. If you are outside running or biking, act like a youngster and run like the wind for a good distance!

It is hard to go wrong with interval training. Just be creative and challenge yourself! Keep in mind that variety is key to quality cardio sessions. Some days you can stick to the "slow and steady" and other days when you feel on top of the world, pick up the pace and see what you are made of with intervals.

People always ask me whether it's better to do low intensity/long duration vs. high intensity/shorter time and I say, DO BOTH! Variety is best for body and mind.

Common Cardio Mistakes

One of the biggest mistakes I notice in the cardio area of a gym is people leaning on the handle bars of the treadmills or step machines. The bars are there for you to use for balance, and if you are new to the machine you should grasp it lightly to make sure you familiarize yourself with it, but *do not* "hang" on so that you can go faster! Hanging on and holding yourself up on the bars will really not do you any good. It may be harder to *not* hold on, but if that is the case then slow the machine down or bring the incline down until you reach a level at which you're capable of working.

I worked with a woman years ago who kept complaining that her neck hurt. I was concerned that it might be from an exercise I had her performing, so I really watched everything she did with me to make sure she was not straining her neck.

One day we were doing some cardio next to one another and I noticed that she was holding herself up on the handle bars of the stair climber with locked arms, and her pace was quite fast. After noticing this, I asked her to bring the pace down and to let go of the bars except for slight balance adjustments. As she did this, she noticed her neck releasing pressure and she actually enjoyed her cardio session.

I firmly believe that you can damage your neck and/or back by not paying attention to proper body positioning. Going faster and hanging on is not going to make the fat come off any faster. Going slower and working harder—on your own—will. I promise!

Another mistake some people make while doing cardio is walking too closely to the treadmill console and bumping their hands on the machine, which will most likely cause them to hold the bars instead of allowing their hands to flow naturally at their sides. If this is *you*, move back on the treadmill and take nice, long strides to keep up with the machine. This will allow you to swing your arms freely without hitting the console.

I know these seem like simple things, but you would be amazed how many people never think about them. When the mistakes are pointed out, people are amazed at the difference in their cardio experience. Remember that the gym does not come with a manual to follow—that's one of the reasons I wrote this book!

Flexibility: Take it Nice and Easy!

I realize that everyone is extremely busy and that stretching doesn't seem important, but let me assure you it is a must and you should, without a doubt, try to fit it in with every workout—even if it is only a few minutes. Stretching will make a world of difference for you mentally and physically.

After I do my warm-up at the gym, I allow a few minutes to stretch the body parts that I am focusing on that session. Likewise at the track, before my sprinting routine begins, I warm up with an easy one-mile jog and then stretch for about 10 minutes. Doing so allows me to completely open up the area that I am going to be working—loosening the joints, ligaments and tendons as well as muscles. Stretching also allows me to mentally focus and keeps my body warm and loose!

Another favorable time to stretch is between weight sets during my 30-60 second rest period. Instead of sitting, I stretch!

Post-workout is another opportune time to get some good stretching in while your body is hot! If you give yourself time to stretch and cool down for 10-15 minutes after an intense workout, your drive home or next appointment will be much more relaxed.

While stretching, concentrate on your breathing, taking deep breaths, inhaling through your nose (for the deepest breath) and then slowly exhaling through your mouth. Proper breathing

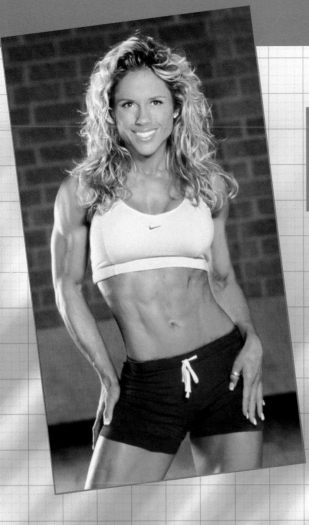

This photo was for an abdominal training article in the Fall 2003 issue of *Muscle & Fitness* magazine.

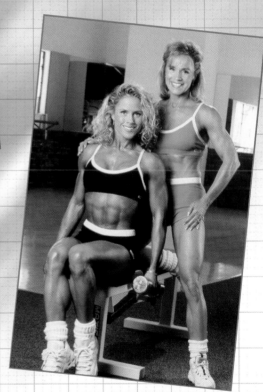

Mom and I posed together for *M&F* when they did a mom/daughter training article in 1998.

Monica Brant

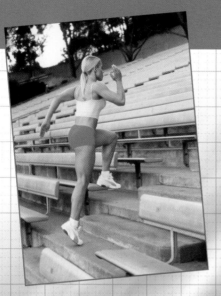

One of the best glute and leg conditioners is stairs! For best results, find a set of them in your area and make a decision to do them one to two times weekly.

Another fun and challenging cardio activity is inline skating. Don't forget to wear your protection!

Photos by Cory Sorensen

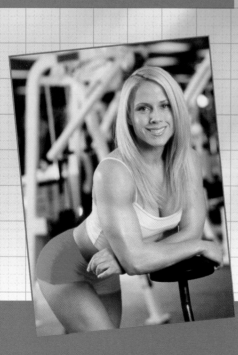

♥ Monica Brant

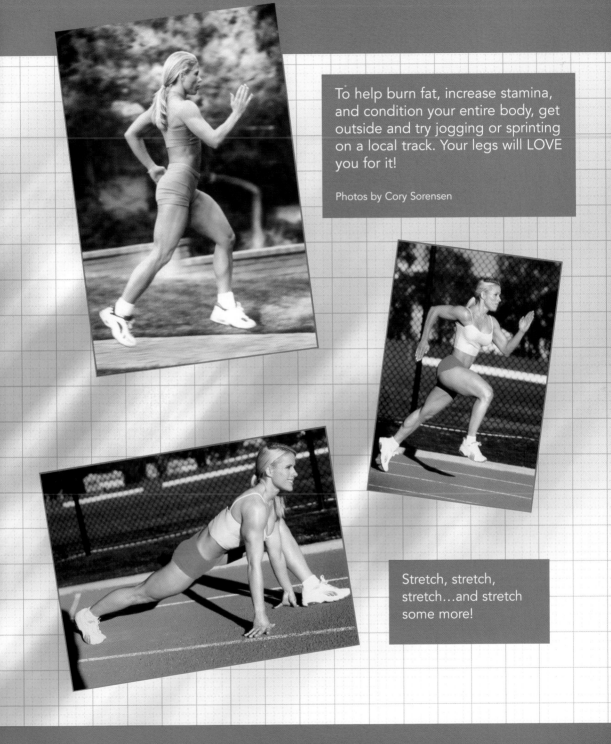

To help burn fat, increase stamina, and condition your entire body, get outside and try jogging or sprinting on a local track. Your legs will LOVE you for it!

Photos by Cory Sorensen

Stretch, stretch, stretch...and stretch some more!

♡ Monica Brant

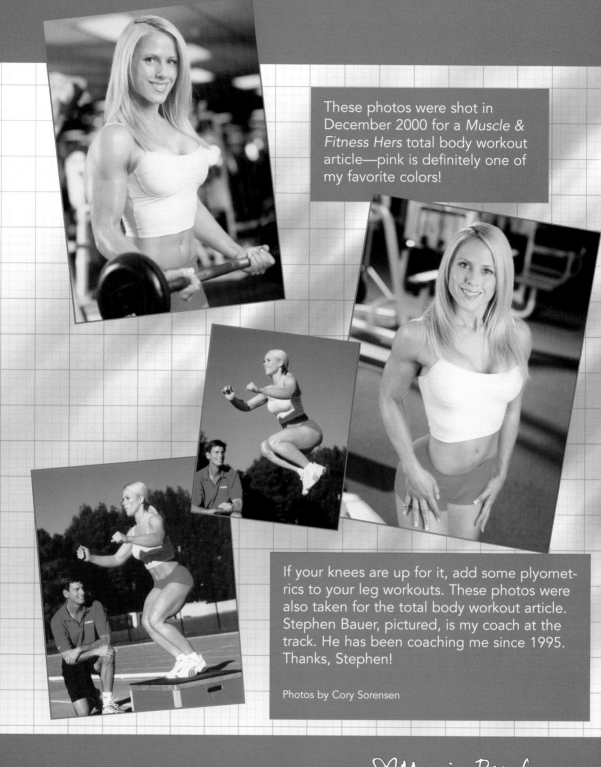

These photos were shot in December 2000 for a *Muscle & Fitness Hers* total body workout article—pink is definitely one of my favorite colors!

If your knees are up for it, add some plyometrics to your leg workouts. These photos were also taken for the total body workout article. Stephen Bauer, pictured, is my coach at the track. He has been coaching me since 1995. Thanks, Stephen!

Photos by Cory Sorensen

♡ Monica Brant

Yes, every so often I do splurge on goodies! Treats are fine as long as they are limited.

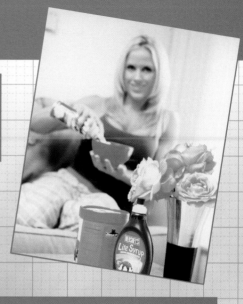

Some of my good ol' standbys: the George Foreman Grill, old-fashioned oatmeal, chicken, veggies, and eggs! These photos were taken for an *M&F Hers* home nutrition/training article in May 2002.

Photos by Cory Sorensen

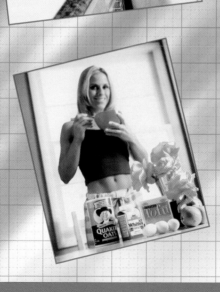

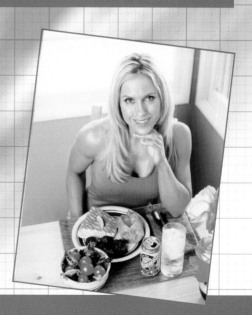

♡ Monica Brant

Oxygen magazine, July 2005. Used with permission.

♡ Monica Brant

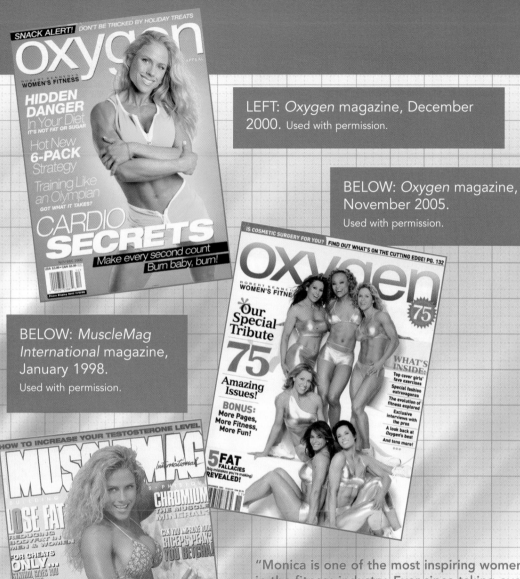

LEFT: *Oxygen* magazine, December 2000. Used with permission.

BELOW: *Oxygen* magazine, November 2005. Used with permission.

BELOW: *MuscleMag International* magazine, January 1998. Used with permission.

"Monica is one of the most inspiring women in the fitness industry. Ever since taking over *Oxygen* magazine almost two years ago, I've yet to meet another person in the business who is as dedicated, hard-working, and truly a pleasure to work with as her. If anyone represents the ever-popular fitness industry it's the fun, fearless Monica Brant."

—Kerrie Lee Brown, editor-in-chief, *Oxygen* magazine

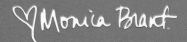

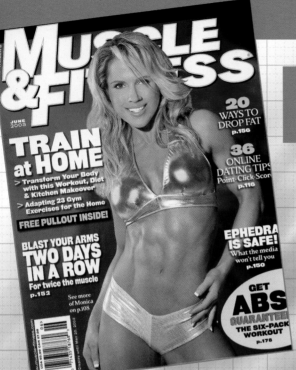

"Monica Brant is unquestionably the top female model in fitness today. For the past decade, she's been the sport's leading spokesperson and most highly photographed individual. A rare combination of charm, grace, beauty and intellect, Monica represents what today's woman is all about."

—Bill Geiger, executive editor, *Muscle & Fitness* magazine

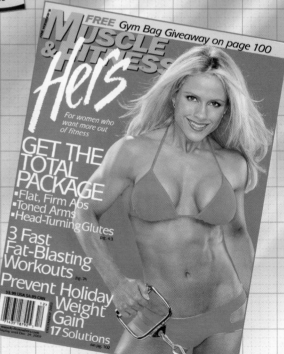

Monica Brant

will help you concentrate on what you are doing and it is also very relaxing! Hold each stretch for approximately 20-30 seconds, without bouncing, at the point where it is uncomfortable but not painful. Sometimes when a muscle is severely tight, I will "massage" the muscle by moving the stretch back and forth in a slow, steady motion. This smooth movement helps lengthen your muscles and extend your stretch.

Keep in mind that as we age we want to be able to lift our arms and do our hair or bend down and put our shoes on. Regular stretching will help you maintain these activities that you might take for granted now.

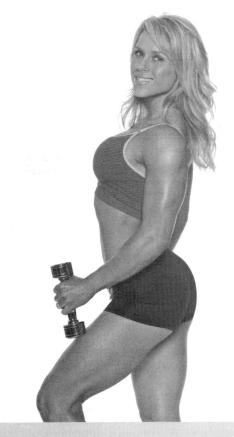

Tips for Success

I have been wearing Polar heart-rate monitors during my cardio sessions for the last 10 years. This allows me to keep my heart rate at the level I need. Not having to stop and try to count my pulse (which has always challenged me!) allows me to have a more effective workout. As long as you are careful not to lose it, it is a one-time investment that will last you for years. You will have to change out the battery from time to time, but that is about it.

Setting the treadmill on a very high incline helps me work my legs and shape my glutes at the same time that I am burning fat. I have found that reading a book while I am on the treadmill makes my cardio time fly by! Remember, at a higher incline my speed is slower and I am able to focus on the book. I have also mastered reading while on the stepmill...but I have yet to learn to read while I am running!

If you are trying to lose inches from your hips (what woman, may I ask, is not? And yes, this includes me!), split your time evenly between cardio and weights. Nutrition is a separate piece of

the puzzle and is probably 80 percent of your success or failure—more on this in the next chapter!

Keep your cardio sessions from becoming boring by switching machines if you are inside the gym. Or, take it outside with a good hike, swim, or sprint. Do stairs or bleachers, run in the sand if you're near a beach, take up inline skating, roller skating, an intense dance class, boxing, kickboxing—anything that keeps your heart going above its resting level and makes you use your body.

Please don't forget how important *rest* is. Resting between exercise sessions is imperative if you want to develop your body and lose the body fat. When we sleep we release growth hormones that help the body repair and recover. (Growth hormones also help to burn fat, since they are also released with exercise.) Do try to get a good night's sleep five to seven times weekly for optimum performance. Some of us need a bit more sleep, and some are fine with less. Find what works best for you personally and then make it happen! Too bad we can't just train, eat, and sleep. We would all be in the best shape!

My Current
Training
Program

In the past few years I have altered my training program several times due to the type of competitions I am involved in. Just a reminder from the "My Story" section—I have been competing in figure competitions since 2003. Upon taking the figure stage, I realized my physique needed some "tweaking" in order to match the requirements of what the IFBB is looking for in the physiques.

For example, at this time I have not trained arms alone for more than two years because it appeared that my arms were muscular enough and that they may have been taking away from my shoulder size. Please keep in mind that I am not recommending this for everyone; I believe that everyone needs to focus on their own body and what it requires.

I feel that my weakest body part is my back. Mentally and physically, I cringe when I have to train back. I am sure this is because I am stronger in the "pushing" movements rather than the "pulling" movements. This is probably also why I enjoy running (pushing off the ground) instead of swimming laps (pulling my body through the water). I have worked specifically on pull-ups for the last couple of years, trying to make my back stronger and wider. Focusing on this difficult exercise helped me mentally too, as I have become strong-er overall. At any rate, my current training schedule is as follows:

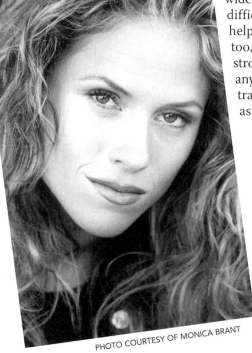

PHOTO COURTESY OF MONICA BRANT

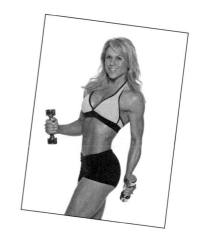

Frequency	Exercise
Monday	Sprints/plyometrics and cardio for 30-60 minutes
Tuesday	Circuit training upper body (chest, shoulders, back, abs; concentrating on shoulders) usually 30-40 minutes, plus cardio lasting 30-60 minutes
Wednesday	Same as Monday
Thursday	Either a day off, if needed, or easy cardio for 30-60 minutes
Friday	Circuit training upper body (chest, shoulders, back, abs; this time concentrating on back) usually 30-40 minutes, plus cardio lasting 30-60 minutes
Saturday	Either sprints/plyometrics or just cardio for 30-60 minutes, or sometimes both depending on how I am feeling and where my body is with regard to when I have to step on stage and how lean I am
Sunday	Circuit training legs and cardio lasting 60-90 minutes

Any day, just for fun, I will add in a dance class at Gold's Gym!

NUTRITION
Chicken
Or Chocolate?

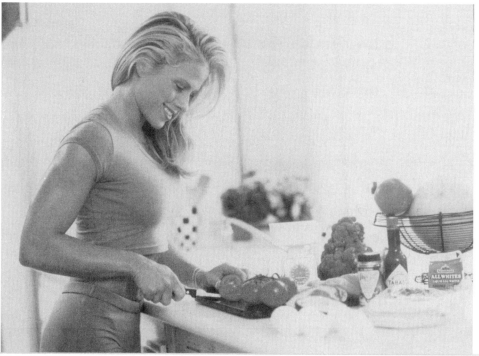

PHOTO BY CORY SORENSEN

Choices—we have to make them every day. We choose what time to get up, whether to hit snooze on the alarm, what to wear, what direction to go to miss traffic, what calls to make, how we will handle stress, whether to smile or to have a bad attitude...the list is endless. With so many things to focus on, why should we add another layer by choosing to eat the best possible foods for our mind, body, and health?

Top 10
Reasons to Eat
Healthfully

I realize most people need lots and lots of reasons to do something different, and that includes changing eating patterns! So to help convince you that healthy eating is worth the effort, I have selected my top 10 reasons why you should start to make the best choices when it comes to food selections. Read on...

1. Choosing to eat healthy *will* increase your mental ability to focus on the tasks at hand and throughout the day, thus allowing you to continue to make other wise choices.

2. Choosing to eat healthy *will* give you the energy to make it through the day with a constant stream of energy, rather than feeling ups and downs as if you're on a roller coaster.

3. Choosing to eat healthy *will* speed up your metabolism so that you will fit into those cute, new jeans. Keep in mind that speeding up your metabolism is a good

thing—can we say "losing fat"? When you choose to eat healthy by combining the proper amounts of macronutrients (protein, carbohydrate, and fat), your body will have to switch "on" its preprogrammed "fast metabolism" mode. There is no way around it. How nice is that? It's something we do not have to think about, for once.

4. Choosing to eat healthy *will* help keep your muscles strong and conditioned. Why go through all the trouble at the gym if you are not going to supply your body with proper nutrition?

5. Choosing to eat healthy *will* increase your bone density (via adequate nutrient intake and providing energy for resistance training), which is very important for us ladies because of our risk of osteoporosis.

6. Choosing to eat healthy *will* increase your confidence, because you are going to look and feel wonderful. I promise. It is so worth it!

7. Choosing to eat healthy *will* help you have more discipline in other areas of your life. Once you master food selections, you can master just about anything else you need to. I call it "controlling the children on your tongue." Those "children," or taste buds, are the reason we want to eat things that typically are not the best choices. Most foods that taste good—the ones we crave—are not foods that will make us feel and look our best. So control those children on your tongue and make them listen to you, the smart one! The healthiest foods are generally those that are hardest to eat all the time, because they can be boring. Of course

there are exceptions to this. For example, a Granny Smith apple tastes pretty good to me—but I can easily think of 100 more exciting and fun-tasting foods.

8. Choosing to eat healthy *will* bolster your immune system, allowing you to better fight infections and to defend against bacteria that you encounter every day.

9. Choosing to eat healthy *will* keep your moods balanced by keeping your blood-sugar levels balanced. Do not be fooled, eating is a very hormonal experience. Insulin is produced by the body, and we all need it to survive. On the other hand, too much insulin leads to fat storage/inhibited fat burning, and increased appetite/hunger. You can avoid excessive amounts of insulin by scrutinizing the amounts of carbohydrates you consume, which will in turn keep your blood-sugar levels steady. Excess insulin also diminishes the release of the hormone glucagon. Glucagon promotes fat burning by inhibiting fat-storing enzymes. Instead, it mobilizes fatty acids from fat stores to be burned for energy. Hooray for glucagon! More on these hormones and what foods trigger them later, when we discuss the macronutrients in detail.

10. Choosing to eat healthy *will* lower your risk of developing countless diseases, from heart disease to hypertension to diabetes to cancer. You'll have a longer, healthier, and happier life!

The Macronutrients: Protein, Carbohydrate and Fat

Protein Power

To function at its best and remain fit, your body requires a substantial amount of protein each and every day! In fact, I believe that protein could be the most important of the three macronutrients. Before we get into the how much and what types, let's take a look at what protein actually is.

Proteins are very large molecules made of amino acids, of which there are approximately 20. About eight of these amino acids are "essential," meaning that they are necessary for life but cannot be synthesized in the body, so you must consume them through food. Every tissue of the body (muscle, hair, skin, nails, etc.) consists of protein. Proteins are also the building blocks of lean muscle tissue. Without protein, BUILDING MUSCLE and BURNING FAT would be IMPOSSIBLE.

Unfortunately, it seems that protein is the most overlooked and under-consumed of all three macronutrients. I find that most people *think* they are eating enough protein, but when I ask them to tell me their day's diet, they respond with,

"Well, today wasn't a good day. I missed breakfast, had a protein bar, ate a bag of chips with a turkey sandwich for lunch, and then went about five hours till I ate a chicken pot-pie."

How Much Protein?

Your first question is probably, "What is the right amount of protein?" Before I go any further, please allow me to remind you that I am *not* a licensed nutritionist, so my advice and opinions solely come from my own experiences. With that in mind, I believe that approximately *0.8 to one gram of protein per pound of bodyweight* is sufficient. That means if you weigh 130 you should try to consume between 104 and 130 grams of protein daily.

I realize this is more than what is often recommended for normal protein intake, but I am basing my assumptions on what I have done with my own intake (and this is why you are reading my book, right?).

Let us also keep in mind that people who are highly active in sports are continually breaking down muscle through exercise and should eat more protein than the average person (hopefully this is you I am describing). If you're dieting it's also important to eat enough protein each day since you are also restricting your calorie intake.

When the body breaks down muscle tissue, it must replace it with something—this is where protein comes into play! If you have not supplied your body with enough protein to feed your muscles, then your body cannot possibly rebuild and strengthen its muscles. The human body has the innate ability to break down muscle tissue for use as an energy source during heavy exercise. This is called "muscle catabolism." *Yucky!* Muscle catabolism can cause muscle soreness, shrinkage of muscle tissue (ever hear of skinny-fat?), and in some cases, lead to injury. This is why it is so important to eat enough protein every

Rounding Out Your Nutrition Plan

Another important factor of a healthy nutrition plan involves your sleeping pattern. We went over the benefits of sleep in the training section, but believe it or not, your sleeping patterns can affect your eating program and how your body functions. Getting plenty of rest is essential to being able to make wise and healthy decisions on your meal plan. These decisions really kick in at night, when we are the most vulnerable to temptation. If you sleep well, you'll wake up with energy and a good attitude about having a productive day.

Speaking of a productive, healthy day, it begins with breakfast. Never skip breakfast! Doing so will cause your body to remain in starvation mode because it is not being relieved of the

"fast" you took overnight. Just because you are sleeping does not mean your body has quit working—and it's working without any energy provided from food. Upon waking, the first thing that will need fuel is your brain, which will be looking for glycogen specifically. If you do not supply your body with food to replace the glycogen, your body will turn to your hard-earned muscle tissue for food. If the only way you'll eat breakfast is by reminding yourself that your muscles will be eaten alive, then by all means think about it like that.

Eating breakfast *will* wake up your metabolism (and you!) and help you control your appetite throughout the day. Be wise and make breakfast your most important meal of the day.

A Day in the Life of Monica's Diet

I like to make my eating plan as simple as possible so that I can maintain it and not have to think too much about what I'm going to eat on a given day. This is a sample of my diet for a typical day:

Meal 1: Protein shake made with water, plus one essential fatty acid gel capsule supplement

Meal 2: Old-fashioned oatmeal made with four egg whites (see my porridge recipe for details)

Meal 3: Four to five ounces buffalo meat, four-ounce potato, ½ cup green beans

Meal 4: Four to five ounces chicken breast, ½ cup rice medley, cucumbers, plus one essential fatty acid gel capsule supplement

Meal 5: Green salad with albacore tuna, topped with low-sugar olive oil and vinegar dressing, and greens (broccoli, broccolini, cucumbers and/or mixed peppers)

Meal 6: Protein shake made with water

This meal plan has worked for me time and again. The constant stream of complex carbs keeps my blood sugar level and maintains my energy. The mixture of proteins supply my muscles with the proper nutrients; I include essential fats for a healthy heart, head, and connective tissue.

At this point I would like to mention that I have worked with nutritionists many times throughout the past decade. I have learned to measure and weigh my food, calculate calories, and keep logs of my eating plans. All of these procedures have taught me about foods, and I have learned how my body responds to different items. I highly suggest that everyone work with an experienced nutritionist at least once in your life. You will learn valuable tools for successful dieting, and you will be accountable to someone other than yourself (which may not be enough to keep you on track).

day to maintain all of the functions for which protein is needed. Also, remember that your body cannot store protein like it can carbohydrates and fats; it is therefore essential that you eat protein with every meal.

I try to consume 120 grams of protein daily. I divide 120 by five or six, depending on how many meals I will be eating that day. If I am up early and stay up late at night, I may try to spread out the meals to six so that I am able to eat every few hours. This means I would need to ingest 20-24 grams of protein per meal. (Six meals x 20 g = 120 g total for the day or five meals x 24 g = 120 g total for day.)

The best ways to find out how many grams are in your proteins are:

• *Learn to read labels*
• *Measure your food*
• *Take notes so that you start recognizing the nutrient content of different items*

The more you research and learn about the foods you eat, the easier it will be for you to successfully follow your diet plan. I realize that measuring your food takes more time, but please remember you are trying to learn, and the only way to do this is by actually going through with it. You need to set that piece of uncooked chicken breast on the scale and see exactly how much it weighs. After a few times of putting it on the scale, you will be able to tell what it weighs just by looking at it, and this will make your protein consumption more efficient. Keep in mind that you can measure meat/poultry/fish after it is cooked, but it will lose about one ounce of weight. (Four ounces of raw chicken will yield approximately three cooked ounces.)

Be sure to purchase all different sizes of measuring spoons and cups and keep them handy to your cooking space. You can also find food scales in different sizes, one for home, one for the office kitchen and one for traveling. Food scales and measuring tools can also be helpful when eating out. I have been known to take my half-cup measuring cup to places such as a Chinese restaurant so that I am not tempted to eat too much rice. Don't be shy! No one is going to seriously care if you are measuring your food (unless you are at a very fancy place—then I might not recommend bringing your measuring cups!) and you never know when you will encourage someone else that may be watching to follow in your healthy-eating footsteps. I believe all of us can help others, and you can be an inspiration to the people around you.

The extra effort of measuring will make a difference for you. Once you have a "good eye" for the weights of different items, it will be much faster to cook and eat. Measuring also goes for carbohydrate and fat items, to be discussed later.

Protein Sources

Proteins can be broken down into different groups based on fat content. Obviously the leaner the protein, the leaner you will become and remain. I try to eat the leanest available proteins most of the time. I occasionally do indulge in some of the higher-fat proteins, salmon being one of my favorites. The following is a list of different types of protein sources.

Very lean protein sources include: skinless white-meat chicken or turkey, flounder, halibut, tuna (fresh or canned in water), lobster, shrimp, clams, fat-free cheese and any meat or cheese with one gram of fat or less per ounce. Egg whites also count as a very lean protein source, as do many whey-based protein powders.

Lean protein sources include: lean beef, lean pork, lean cuts of lamb or veal, skinless dark-meat chicken, sardines, salmon, tuna (canned in oil) and any meat or cheese with approximately two or three grams of fat per ounce.

Medium-fat protein sources include: most beef products, dark-meat chicken with skin, fried chicken or fried fish, and any meat or cheese with approximately five grams of fat per ounce like regular pork, lamb or veal. Eggs fit into this category, as well.

High-fat protein sources include: pork spareribs, pork sausage, bacon, regular cheese, processed sandwich meat and any meat or cheese with approximately eight or more grams of fat per ounce.

It will be important for you to research the amount of protein per ounce of your selections. It's necessary to take the time to read labels if you are going to track your protein intake.

For example, one large egg will equal three grams of protein per white and three grams of protein per yolk, so if you have four scrambled egg whites at breakfast, that only equals 12 grams of protein. One four-ounce chicken breast at lunchtime will net you 24 grams of protein, making your total for the day 36 grams of protein. You can see that to get to 80 grams or more, you would need a few more excellent sources of protein.

It's very difficult to get to 100 grams (or more) of protein daily. That's one reason I usually have protein shakes, which are convenient sources of high-quality protein (more on this later). Another thing to keep in mind is that a high protein intake usually also increases your fat intake, unless you are extremely careful in selecting and preparing your protein sources.

If possible, I prefer to alternate my proteins with each meal. For example, on any given day, I might include the following different items:

- *Protein shake*
- *Egg whites/egg (you can have a whole egg once or twice per day)*
- *Buffalo or other lean steak*
- *Chicken*
- *Fish*

I think variety is best nutritionally and mentally. It will be much easier for you to stick to your healthy diet if you eat different foods throughout the day.

I realize I have not addressed milk and dairy products; this is mainly because I do not eat them unless I am having a dessert or enjoying pizza. (Oops...did I say that?) I am not going to go into a lot of chatter about my competitions, but when I am trying to get down to 7% body fat for the stage, one of the last things I should do is have any dairy products.

For the most part, dairy products do include good protein, but the problem is that they also are laden with fat (like cheese) or sugar (like yogurt). To actually eat enough dairy to make much of a difference in my protein amounts, I would have to ingest too much of the fat and sug-

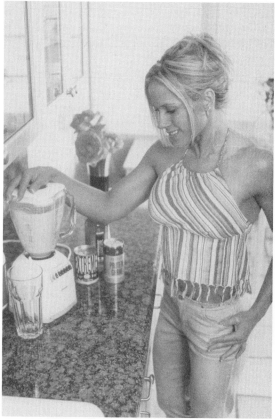

PHOTO BY CORY SORENSEN

ars. Of course there are fat-free cheeses available, but I find them unappetizing and therefore unfulfilling. If I am going to eat cheese, I will eat a very small amount of the real thing. Of course, weighing cheese will help keep you honest when adding it to your egg omelet.

Dairy products are usually high in calcium, which is definitely important. If you choose to limit your dairy intake due to allergies, tolerance problems or any other reason, be sure you take a calcium supplement or choose non-dairy calcium-rich foods. Check with a doctor to see how much calcium you should be getting.

One of the easiest ways to track your food intake and also keep yourself accountable is by keeping a journal of what you eat. It could look something like the sample meal plan shown below.

The amount of food equals 128 grams of protein, which could be perfect for your body type and activity level. As long as you go to bed before 10 p.m., you could be just fine. But if you are like me (and I am sure many of you are) there are too many things to do in a day and not enough hours to do them, which means you end up staying up later than planned and become hungry again—*Grrrrr.*

At this point I recommend having another protein shake, egg-white omelet or possibly a lean cut of red meat (such as London Broil) to help keep you satiated while you sleep. I find that if I go to bed too hungry I will wake up and not be able to get back to sleep until I have something to eat. This not only leads to eating something you really should not eat in the middle of the night, but it also disrupts your much-needed rest.

What About Whey?

As I mentioned earlier, I frequently drink whey protein shakes to bump up my protein amount and keep my metabolism moving. In case you are unfamiliar with this great product, let me introduce to you to one of the best forms of complete protein. Whey is a byproduct of the cheese-making process. It contains all essential and non-essential amino acids and has the highest form of concentrations of branched chain amino acids (BCAAs) found in nature.

Studies have found that whey may reduce cancer rates by protecting the body from carcinogens, improve immuni-

(continued on page 68)

Sample Meal Plan

Day 1: Monday		Protein (g)	Carbohydrate (g)	Fat (g)
6:30 a.m.	protein shake w/ water	25	1	1.5
9:30 a.m.	4 egg whites, 1 yolk, 1/2 cup oats	15	27	3
12:45 p.m.	4 oz. chicken breast, 1/2 cup rice, steamed green beans, 1 1/2 ounces of slivered almonds on greens	37	38	28
4:00 p.m.	protein shake w/ water	25	1	1.5
7:30 p.m.	halibut, green salad with 1/2 tbsp olive oil and vinegar, 2-3 oz. red potato	26	15	10

Sample Daily Meal Journal   DATE: _____

Meal 1 (list all foods/drinks):	# PROTEIN grams	# CARB grams	# FAT grams
Meal 2 (list all foods/drinks):			
Meal 3 (list all foods/drinks):			
Meal 4 (list all foods/drinks):			
Meal 5 (list all foods/drinks):			
Meal 6 (list all foods/drinks):			
	PROTEIN	CARBS	FATS
TOTAL GRAMS			
	Multiply X 4	Multiply X 4	Multiply X 9
TOTAL CALORIES			

ADD TOGETHER THE TOTAL MACRONUTRIENT CALORIES
TO GET YOUR **TOTAL DAILY CALORIES**

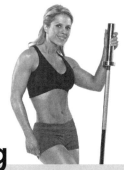

Calorie Counting

To count or not to count? This can be a very confusing area for many and it can take up much valuable time. However, I do feel that it is important to understand how to make calories work for your body. One of my first nutritionists taught me how to keep track of my calories by keeping a journal of my meals and the breakdown of each meal specifically regarding amounts of carbohydrate, protein and fat. This way at the end of the day I could see if I made my calorie target for the day.

When I was competing in Fitness I followed a meal plan that would allow me up to 2,000 calories per day. I realize that seems like a lot of calories, and it is, but for the type of intense exercise I was doing for competitions I had to get the nutrition to supply my body with constant energy and macronutrients for recovery. It is extremely hard to eat that much (healthy) food and it takes lots of preparation and discipline. This is where the journal was helpful for me. I could see the calories adding up for the day and it would give me encouragement to consume the proper amounts. I am a visual person, and seeing the numbers on the paper really helped keep my focus.

At this point in my life I do not need to eat as many calories since my competitions are not as physically challenging. Of course, I still focus on eating the proper ratio of macronutrients (especially when preparing for a contest), which for me is approximately 35% protein, 45% carbohydrate and 20% fat. Remember, you have to eat to lose fat!

I don't give specific calorie recommendations here because I don't think you can accurately determine what your body needs with a one-size-fits-all equation. For tailored advice I really recommend going to a nutritionist who can determine the amount of calories your body needs to lose, gain, or maintain weight.

In addition, even if you determine that you should be eating 1,800 calories daily, it's very difficult (if not impossible) to accurately count calories. To truly add everything up correctly, you will have to be incredibly strict and diligent, record every morsel you eat or drink, then use an accurate calorie-counting program or book to calculate your intake. If you eat at restaurants it's almost impossible to accurately determine the amount of calories in your meal.

One other way to determine a rough guide of the calories you should be taking in is by doing the opposite approach. For three representative days (don't do this on Thanksgiving or your birthday), record everything you eat and drink and the amounts of your servings. Then calculate your intake for each day, add it all up, and divide by three to get your daily average intake. Say you get an average of 2,000 calories and you want to lose a few pounds. You can slash 10-15% off of that number, so that you instead strive to eat 1,700 to 1,800 calories daily.

A few words of caution: Don't drop below 1,200 calories daily, and don't think that fewer calories is better. If you drop too low, your body will instead go into "starvation mode" where it slows its metabolic rate and refuses to burn fat efficiently, causing the "skinny-fat" syndrome.

Another approach is to make protein consumption your number-one goal. You do need to count your protein grams (see the calculations in the protein section). Then add in a few servings of starchy carbs and healthy fat, and vegetables should cover the rest. If you don't want to count calories, I really recommend counting your protein grams (at least in the beginning) to ensure you're meeting your goal of approximately 0.8 to 1 gram per pound of your bodyweight.

ty, reduce stress and lower cortisol (a hormone responsible for some fat storing due to high stress levels), combat HIV, increase brain serotonin levels, reduce blood pressure, and improve physical performance. Plus, whey protein can speed up your metabolism, which will help you burn fat.

As you can see, whey is an excellent protein source and should be considered a "must-have" of proteins. Keep in mind that not all whey protein powders are the same. In my opinion the "isolate" or "concentrates" are the highest form of whey powders. There is so much research done on whey proteins, let me suggest that you take some time one day and do your own studies on the subject to further your understanding. One more thing—as you'll see in the "traveling tips" section, most whey protein powders are easily mixable with water, so it is a great source of on-the-go nutrition.

To summarize protein choices, the leaner someone eats, the leaner her body will be. Variety is best for physical and mental health, yes, but the bulk of your protein should come from lean sources. Of course, avoiding high-fat proteins is best all the way around—not only for leanness but also for the heart and arteries.

Carbohydrates:
A Complex Issue

The next macronutrient of interest is carbohydrate, commonly referred to as "carbs." Carbs have become very confus-

ing for people, mostly because of popular diet books. Some say to eat more carbs while others say to eat little to no carbs. In my (humble) opinion and from my experience, carbs are necessities in the human body. They supply energy to your muscles and to your brain. How are you going to manage to get through all the daily decisions you have to make without having fuel for your brain?

I like to divide carbohydrates into two broad categories: simple and complex. You'll find many different categories of carbohydrates, but I like to think of simple carbs as sugar sources such as fruit-flavored yogurt, honey, bananas, and fat-free cookies. These hit your blood system rapidly and increase your insulin levels just as quickly (remember what we said about insulin levels and fat absorption earlier?). They provide your body and brain with immediate energy and also enable the body to store fat rapidly. If you do not use

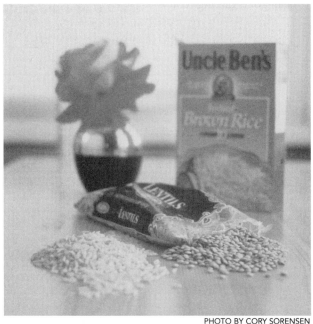

PHOTO BY CORY SORENSEN

them right away, they will decide to make your thighs home and cause you to become sleepy at all the wrong times once your blood sugar level drops.

Simple carbs may sound scary, but they can actually have positive effects on your body if you eat them at the appropriate times. One of the best times to take in simple carbs is immediately following an intense training routine. (For post-workout recovery, see the Ask Monica section.) You'll then be on your way to a better body by supplying your muscles with lost glycogen, which aids in recuperation time and lean muscle production.

Complex carbs, on the other hand, have more of a "timed-release" action, making them the choice of champions in the carb category. Eating complex carbs throughout the day will help keep your glucose (blood sugar) levels stable and help you feel alert throughout the day.

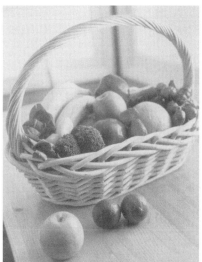

PHOTO BY CORY SORENSEN

Don't be afraid to eat complex carbs in the afternoon or evening, especially if you are going to be up late or have an important paper (or book!) to write and will be needing brainpower. By cutting the amounts of that particular serving in half, you won't have any carbohydrate left over for your hips and thighs!

Complex carbs are also commonly referred to as starches, including bread, potatoes and rice. These carbs enter the bloodstream more slowly. This brings us to the glycemic index (GI), a graph show-casing all carbs and the rate at which they enter the bloodstream when consumed. It is important to have a good grasp on the GI and to know approximately where your favorite carbs fall on the index. (For foods other than what are described here, you can find a complete list in a nutrition book or on the web.)

A food's glycemic index number only gives you the information from that food being consumed alone, without any other macronutrients. The rate of absorption will change somewhat if you consume the given food with other selections. In general, carbs that break down quickly during digestion have the highest glycemic index ratings, whereas carbs that break down slowly (releasing glucose gradually into the bloodstream) have lower numbers.

The higher GI carbohydrates are absorbed into the bloodstream more quickly, and thus inhibit your fat-burning ability faster. Not all complex carbs have a low GI level. For instance, rice cakes, instant rice, white potatoes and most white breads have the highest levels. Old-fashioned oatmeal, whole-grain rye bread, sweet potatoes, apples, and whole-wheat pasta have a medium absorption rate. The lowest on the totem pole of the GI are soybeans, almonds, peanuts and walnuts. However, these low-GI foods are high in fat, which lead to an increase in overall caloric level. You will be surprised to find that some

Troubleshooting Problems: What if it isn't working?

I often hear complaints that someone's diet just isn't working, that the fat just isn't coming off and "Please help me!" Everyone wants a simple solution and fortunately there is one, but it's not necessarily easy. Being successful with your diet is a big problem; it can even be a problem for me at times too, especially when I am not preparing for a contest. It appears to me that many people just do not understand how hard it really is to:

1. Commit to a healthy eating plan at all times, and;

2. Be patient enough with the plan to allow your body to change.

If you're not blessed with an amazing metabolism and genetics, chances are your body does not want to be lean…it desperately wants to stay full-figured! Obviously there's nothing wrong with being full-figured, but for many of us, it just doesn't cut it. I prefer the way I feel and look when I am leaner.

Though I have to get very lean for competitions, I prefer to be around 11-12% body fat. The general public's view of a woman's proper body fat percentage is somewhere around 18-22% percent, which is much higher than I like to be. After years of competing professionally and seeing myself in photos, I have a very set mind of how I want to look at all times. This doesn't mean that it is easy for me or that it doesn't take *constant* work—because it does. Every day I have to make certain choices to maintain the way I look (or should I say every night, as night time is when it is harder for me to be good!).

If you are trying to troubleshoot your fat-loss problem, my advice is to go back to the basics and consider what you have been feeding your body for the last few days or weeks. Start writing down your eating habits and make yourself be accountable to the calories you are ingesting. When I do this, I typically find one of the following three scenarios:

- I'm not taking in enough total calories
- I'm eating too many of the wrong items
- I'm not eating enough carbs throughout the day, which in turn causes me to crave starchy carbs in the evening when I am less likely to be strong

When you write down each item that goes into your mouth, you'll most likely notice that your food selections could improve. You might also notice that you aren't eating enough times in a day, and/or that you aren't consuming enough calories. Your body has to have enough calories just to maintain itself—in addition to its duties of repair and recovery from long hours of work and exercise.

(continued on page 71)

---

healthy foods (potatoes, for example) have a higher GI rating than some less-healthy foods (ice cream, for example).

The GI is a learning tool for you, regarding how carbohydrates affect your glucose level. It is not the "be all, end all," and should be viewed as a tool in your toolbox of knowledge for better understanding of foods.

The last important carb source is good ol' fibrous carbs. Fibrous carbs fall under the complex category, and are high in fiber, nutrients, and water.

My motto is "Green is Good!" Most anything green and crunchy is good to munch on, including lettuce, spinach, green beans, cucumbers, broccoli, celery and zucchini. You can just about never eat too much of these.

Most people do not eat enough vegetables, so I suggest that you eat them any time you like—just get them in. These produce items are extremely helpful in the evenings when you might be hungry and do not want to add extra calories, but need to eat something. The veggies will help fill your belly so that you can rest easy knowing you are not producing lots of unwanted fat.

Favored Fats

Let's start with what I like to call the *ugly* fats, which are broken down into two categories: saturated and hydrogenated. Saturated fats are generally solid at room temperature and come mostly from animal sources. Some examples of saturated fats are butter, lard, and fat on a steak, but remember that saturated fats can also be found in chocolate bars and fried foods such as potato chips. Saturated fats can

Troubleshooting Problems (cont.)

We don't usually remember how many meals we have missed or how many of the wrong selections we have made—then we wonder why we're not seeing more results. We all pretend that small bag of Cheetos or the Kit-Kat chocolate bar doesn't really count—that we ate it early enough and did enough cardio to burn it off! We forget that each day counts and we forget about all the small bites of this and that, which all add up. Do not think for one minute that your body is going to take those calories and say, "Oh! Look what we have here: 500 grams of carbs and 150 grams of fat. Why don't I just get rid of it for my owner?"

No, our bodies say something more like this, "Oh! Look what we have here: 500 grams of carbs and 150 grams of fat. I should store this in a very safe spot, let's say on the stomach, to protect the ovaries and how about some on the glutes so when my nice owner sits down, she will be more comfortable with the cushion!"

Everything you put in your mouth can and will be used for either good or bad purposes. When you are not seeing results, it is often because you are adding little extras but aren't keeping track of them.

Of course there are times when our bodies hit plateaus even when we *are* eating properly and effectively. At that point I recommend again going through your eating plan and possibly adding some more good-quality calories (more meaning maybe 200 per day, not 600). It could be that you have been eating a medium amount of calories and now your metabolism is running faster. I would definitely suggest not changing all aspects of your diet and training at once. You will need to do one thing at a time to see exactly what you are missing.

If the extra calories don't stimulate your body to let go of the fat, tweak your training program. Up your cardio and/or intensity level or start lifting heavier weights for three to six weeks. No, you won't become a huge bodybuilder overnight from lifting heavier weights! Remember that weights will help you develop your muscles and burn fat.

The process of fat loss and maintenance is constant and will continue to change depending on your weight, age, genetic makeup, and of course, determination. It can't be something you do for a couple weeks and then abandon, especially if you have been heavy most of your life. It will take some extra time to teach your body to be comfortable at each new body fat level. Be patient with yourself, but also be diligent to constantly challenge yourself each day.

Let me also remind you that if you have never hired an experienced nutritionist before, now would be a good time to do so. It's amazing what you can achieve with the proper guidance and support. The nutritionist will help you develop a routine that you can follow and will then make adjustments as necessary. This will eliminate most of the guessing game for you and you'll have someone to whom you are accountable.

The eating patterns that you need to take, and keep, the fat off are simple, but challenging, due to our hectic lives and daily emotional struggles. If you're aware of this and can clearly think through your decisions, you will find you can make permanent changes.

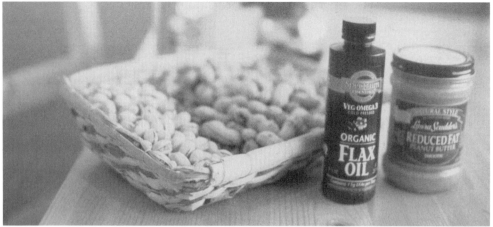

increase insulin resistance and inhibit fat burning.

Hydrogenated fats are derived from an artificial process that makes them more stable and harder at room temperature. Shortening and margarine are two examples, along with many packaged foods (cookies/crackers) that contain "partially hydrogenated vegetable oil." Such partially hydrogenated oils are a source of "trans fats," which you definitely want to limit. Trans fats can increase your cholesterol levels and increase your risk for heart disease. These fats are definitely *not* essential!

I know that foods like cookies, chips and crackers taste good; you even crave these "comfort foods" at times! Just do yourself a huge favor and save them for the time when you really feel you deserve them. One trick I try to do before or after eating something of the sort is to drink a whey protein shake (made only with water) along with the item of choice. This will help your body fight off the insulin rush that the "goodie" will cause. Again, I highly suggest you limit your intake of these fats to the bare minimum.

If you are wondering exactly what would be on the list of saturated/hydrogenated fats, here is a list of common items to either avoid if possible or, at the least, limit:

- *Fatty cuts of beef*
- *Hamburger*
- *Bacon*
- *Sausage*
- *Organ meats*
- *Poultry skin*
- *Margarine*
- *Solid shortening*
- *Cream*
- *Whole milk*
- *Most cheeses*
- *Full-fat cream cheese*
- *Full-fat sour cream*
- *Egg yolks*
- *Most chips and all fried foods*
- *Any foods made with palm and/or coconut oils*
- *Chocolate bars (Oh, don't hate me for this one)*

If you have to eat something off this list, please use extreme caution and try eating only half a serving or less of the

Traveling Tips

I travel frequently, sometimes every weekend for months at a time. I always try to take a few meals with me when traveling so that I am never caught without food. This is especially important when I am preparing for a competition. If I'm preparing for a competition, packing my food is almost more important than packing my makeup. Packing for a trip *always* includes packing meals. I've learned that if I take it with me, I'm less tempted by the fast food and goodies sold at the airports. This saves some money, too.

Here are my ideas to simplify on-the-go eating, whether you're traveling out of town or just to work for the day!

- **Tuna is one of the easiest** choices when it comes to packing and carrying. You can take a couple cans or pouches of tuna for each day you will be gone to ensure you will have at least 20-45 grams of readily available protein. You can eat it alone or have it with some salad, which you can find at just about any fast-food restaurant. I realize that not everyone likes the smell of tuna so if you open it on a plane or in a closed car you may upset your neighbor. I have done both, so I am speaking from experience! Since the cans are heavier and contain less protein (19 grams), I prefer the pouches (23 grams) even though they are slightly more expensive. The pouches are much easier to open as you don't have to drain them, plus they won't weigh your luggage down. I typically carry a plastic baggie with me so I can dispose of the pouch or can. (If you are at home, be sure to rinse the container before throwing it in the trash.) I know these tips seem obvious, but it never hurts to have easier methods of keeping things clean...and tuna smells up the place so quickly!

- **Celery makes a great snack** to go along with tuna. The crunchiness helps with that "gotta-have-crunch" feeling, and celery's watery aspect makes the tuna dissolve better when chewing. Celery is pretty easy to carry, too. Just chop some up and store it in a baggie.

- **Another quick protein travel tip** is to measure your protein powder into small snack-size baggies, each enough for one shake. Like the tuna, I will also pack one or two baggies of protein powder for each day I'll be gone. I can then quickly grab one bag and mix it up with water, or blend it if a blender is handy. Most whey protein has "stir" ability, which means you can stir it quite easily in some water with a fork or spoon (without blending) and quickly get a smooth consistency.

- **If your work has a kitchen** or break room available for employees, be sure to invest in a small blender that you can leave there. A quick protein shake in between meetings is a great pick-me-up and will help you get in the water you should be drinking—hydration is very important for concentration.

As long as you are not allergic to nuts, I suggest having a small handful after having your tuna or protein shake. Notice that I said *after*. Eating the nuts beforehand will most likely cause you to eat more than you really need; eating them afterward should help you have some discipline.

(continued on page 76)

item. If you can master this "half only" rule, then you can master anything regarding your eating plan.

Next up are polyunsaturated fats, which are better for your body compared to saturated and trans fats. Polyunsaturated fats can affect your cholesterol levels negatively (by lowering "healthy" HDL cholesterol in addition to lowering "lousy" LDL cholesterol), but they are definitely "heart healthier" than saturated or trans fats. These fats do add *calories* to your diet quickly as all fat grams count for nine calories per gram (as compared to protein and carbs, which are only four calories per gram). Polyunsaturated fats are found in most vegetable oils such as canola, soybean, sunflower and safflower. They are generally liquid at room temperature.

Monounsaturated fats are the most desirable, as they lower "lousy" cholesterol, but leave the "healthy" HDL cholesterol levels alone. Olive oil is the most commonly known of these fats. Monounsaturated sources also include canola oil, pecans, almonds, and avocados. (Most fats such as canola oil contain two or all three types of fats.) Monounsaturated fats make up a large part of the Mediterranean-type diet that is thought to lower risk of heart disease. Finally, a good fat that we can enjoy!

One special category of fats is called "essential fatty acids." These actually come from polyunsaturated sources and there are two main types: omega-6 and omega-3. Omega-6 fatty acids are the more commonly consumed; they come from vegetable oils like corn, sunflower, and safflower. In general, Americans need to increase their intake of omega-3s, which come from canola and flaxseed oil, soybean products, and walnuts. Special kinds of omega-3 fats are EPA (eicosapentaenoic acid) and DHA (docosahexaenoic acid), which are found in fish oils from salmon, mackerel, sardines and more.

In place of chicken at some of your meals, I highly recommend substituting three to four ounces of salmon. This will supply 20-26 grams of protein and a great supply of omega-3 fats. One of my favorite treats while dieting is to go to dinner somewhere such as Outback Steakhouse and order the grilled salmon with steamed broccoli. I usually have half of the salmon fillet left over and can eat it the following day for an extra bonus. If you don't eat fish, you will be able to gain the benefits from omega-3 fatty acids from plant sources such as walnuts, flax oil and canola oil.

Keeping Fat Under Control

It's very important to measure oils and other sources of fat—one tablespoon typically equals 14 grams of fat or 126 fat calories. Do not be timid about using your cute little measuring spoon when you are out having a salad with oil and vinegar so that you can keep an eye on your oil dose. Go all out with the vinegar if you like, but try to limit the fat to just one tablespoon. I like to put the oil on first and then the vinegar; it will help spread the oil out over your salad. I like to include healthy fats two to three times per day, but remember to keep your servings small.

To summarize, most of your fat sources should come from olive oil, canola oil, nuts, seeds and fish. Limit sources such as butter, red meat, whole milk, regular cheese and anything that says "partially hydrogenated vegetable oil" on the package.

What To Drink

What About Water?

Water is by far the most abundant substance in our bodies (more than 65% of your body is water), which means our bodies absolutely need water, every day and all the time. We should be constantly supplying ourselves with water—at least eight full glasses a day. I believe if you are exercising, you probably could use even more. I realize that many women don't like to drink throughout the day as it causes you to run to the ladies room, but without proper amounts of water your body will become dehydrated.

Drinking plenty of water can only be beneficial for you. Let me share with you the positive aspects of drinking water so you will start reaching for that bottle (of water!) more often.

- *Drinking water is obviously vital for life. Period.*

- *Drinking water encourages fat burning and muscle growth.*

- *Drinking water helps to lubricate the joints, increasing mobility.*

- *Drinking water can reduce food cravings and helps control appetite.*

- *Drinking water rids your body of water retention (bloating).*

- *Drinking water helps rid the body of toxins and waste.*

- *Drinking water helps your digestive system. It's up to you to keep your intestines "wet enough" so that they can do their job properly by digesting smoothly and eliminating waste.*

- *Drinking water helps control your body temperature. How thirsty are you after an intense workout where you are sweating a lot?*

So just face the fact that you will be making trips to the ladies room, but think of it as adding extra steps to your day that will in turn burn more calories. Yay! Oh, maybe your ladies room is upstairs, and then you can take the stairs too!

What Else to Drink?

Other than water, you can consume a moderate amount of other beverages such as tea, coffee, and diet sodas, but keep in mind that each of them has some negative side effects. I personally think that drinking less of these products will enhance your health and add years to your life.

With regard to caffeine (which, along with nicotine and alcohol, is one of the most widely used mood-affecting drugs in the world), recent studies have proven it to be more negative on the body than positive. Though some studies show that caffeine can stimulate the metabo-

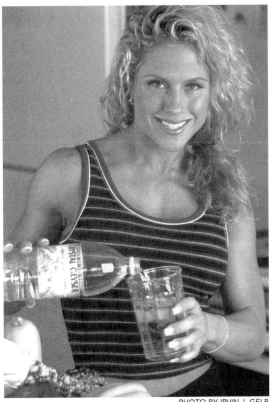

PHOTO BY IRVIN J. GELB

lism by mobilizing fatty acids so that they can be burned for energy, I believe that the negative side effects far outweigh the positive.

Caffeine can affect the length and quality of your sleep. Heavy caffeine users suffer from sleep deprivation, because their nervous system is too stimulated to allow them deep, restful or prolonged sleep. A high intake can also result in a jittery feeling, with shaking hands, palpitations, and wobbliness in the legs.

Unfortunately, for those of you who are addicted to caffeine and feel it is time to reduce your levels, you will have some minor withdrawal discomforts. These include headaches, lethargy, drowsiness, irritability, trembling, restlessness, and reduced concentration. As with any

(continued on page 79)

Traveling Tips (cont.)

• **I will also take oatmeal with me,** measuring 1/2 cup (one serving) into a small baggie along with one packet of Splenda. I bring one bag for each day I'll be gone. Almost every hotel I have stayed at has a coffee maker or microwave available in the room, so I can cook the oatmeal or at least mix it with hot water. Call ahead to confirm and/or request one if you are unsure. You can easily make oatmeal in your room for breakfast—this way you save some money on room service and can make sure of the amount and content of your oatmeal. Some restaurants make it with milk and almost always give you way more than you need...just another temptation if you like oatmeal for breakfast.

For something different, you can mix your pre-measured protein powder (I typically mix one part vanilla and one part chocolate protein powders together) in with your oats after you cook them. If you have access to a coffee maker, you can heat the water, pour it over the oats/protein mix and stir. You will only need about a 1/2 cup of water; I suggest adding a small amount of water and mixing well—you can always add more if needed. If you do not have a coffee maker in the hotel room, ask room service to bring some hot water up! Along with the oats and protein powder, I sometimes add a packet of Splenda and some natural almond butter. I typically carry (or pack) a small Tupperware container with a spoon. (Sometimes I bring two containers if I anticipate needing two on-the-go meals.) This little concoction almost tastes like

chocolate-oatmeal cookie dough! Okay, maybe not that good, but we can pretend...right?

• **Another easy carb source** I have found is Brown Rice Snaps, in baked, unsalted, and Tamari sesame-flavored varieties. They are exceptional and make the tuna pretty easy to handle. They are gluten-free for those of you who can't have wheat, and nine crackers have only 13 grams of carbs, no sugar and just half a gram of fat. Since they don't contain oils or preservatives, you must keep them airtight after opening. These are great snacks with peanut butter or almond butter on top. The brand I like is called Edward & Sons and it's available at health-food stores.

Whatever you decide to take along, be sure to plan ahead and pack the essentials. You will want to keep your immune system as high as possible while traveling, so be sure to keep taking any vitamins you regularly take and keep your food as similar as possible to what you eat at home. These small things should help your body stay healthy. If you are flying, definitely take a couple small bottles of water with you; if you finish those on the flight, ask the flight attendant for more. Drinking as much as you can will help eliminate water retention, which is almost unavoidable when flying. Be sure to watch your sodium and sugar intake prior to flying as well—those too will make your body hold water. Depending on what shoes you wear, you may not be able to wear them after you fly if you don't pay attention to your sodium and water intake.

Smart Shopping

Grocery shopping can be scary, especially if you are hungry. Under no circumstances should you enter a grocery store hungry! Besides having the urge to dive into a box of Mrs. Field's White Chocolate Macadamia Nut Cookies (okay, I have revealed my favorite cookies), you may lack the ability to fight the temptations that lurk on every aisle of the store.

The best way to fight the temptations of food shopping is to eat something prior to going to the store. You can also carry your prepared meal into the store and eat while cruising around the outer aisles. (Most of the staple ingredients of a healthy diet are on the outer aisles, so that's where you'll spend most of your time.)

Aside from eating before shopping, having a list saves time and helps me avoid buying tempting foods. If I go into the grocery store with my list handy and a pen ready to check off the items I add to the cart, I will be out of the tempting store faster and less likely to fall off the wagon. Developing a healthy shopping list is essential to having a good experience in the store. Make no mistake—if you purchase a tempting food, you are much more likely to eat it than if you do not buy it in the first place. Healthy eating begins (and almost ends) with the purchasing process.

I will typically try to purchase the same items at the store each time so that I know exactly what I will eat at home. Since my schedule is usually very full, I do not have extra minutes to spend wondering what I am going to eat. For me, it's most convenient to purchase the same items and eat (mostly) the same things every day.

Try using the list provided here to fill your shopping cart smartly.

Smart Shopping List

Protein Sources
Eggs
Reduced-fat cheddar or mozzarella cheese
Non-fat cottage cheese
Tofu
Chicken, turkey, lean red meat
Unsweetened, plain soymilk
Low-sugar, plain yogurt

Starchy Carbohydrate Sources
Old-fashioned oatmeal
Cream of Rice
Cream of Wheat
Corn tortillas
English muffins
Vogel brand flax and soy bread (you can find Vogel bread in health-food stores and some grocery stores)
Natural granola (pick the brand with the least amount of sugar)
Cereal (pick cereal that is low in sugar and high in fiber)
Potatoes (small red potatoes work great—they are already small so you can eat the whole thing)
Corn
Yellow squash

Fibrous Carbohydrate Sources
Most of the items I have on the fibrous list are green. My motto for veggies is "Green is Good." Keep this in mind when you are shopping for your veggies.

Spinach
Green beans
Lettuce (Butter lettuce is my favorite. Purchasing bagged lettuce will make eating salad more enjoyable, unless you enjoy chopping up lettuce and have the time to do so.)
Broccoli
Broccolini (This is a combination of broccoli and kale. It has a sweeter taste than broccoli alone.)
Broccoli sprouts
Green onions
Cucumbers
Zucchini
Green/red/yellow peppers (I like to purchase the pre-cut and mixed packages, which make salad prep easier. If it's easier, I will eat it at home more readily.)
Celery

Smart Shopping List (cont.)

Fruit Sources
- Green apples (These have less sugar than red apples.)
- Grapefruit
- Bananas (Just eat a third of a large banana at a time, or half of a small banana.)
- Strawberries (These are naturally high in sugar, so limit yourself to only 2-3 medium-sized berries in the morning.)
- Cantaloupe and honeydew melons (Limit to a quarter of a melon in the morning to avoid too much sugar at once.)

Fat Sources
- Nuts, including walnuts, almonds, peanuts, pecans and cashews
- Avocados
- Natural peanut butter
- Natural almond butter
- Flaxseed oil
- Olive oil
- Safflower oil

Preparation is Key

You should prepare as much of your food as you can prior to the day you'll eat it. This will increase your chances of making the best choices for your daily meals and ensure that you won't skip any meals.

You have to plan ahead to stay on track—you can't allow yourself room to ask, "What's to eat?" If you already know what you will eat and your food is already prepared, you'll be able to stay ahead of your cravings. Schedule a "shopping" day each week (or if you have room for plenty of food in your freezer, it can be once every two weeks) so you always have enough food at hand to prepare.

I like to buy the large or family-size containers of skinless, boneless chicken breasts. Once home I will immediately put on some latex disposable gloves, plug in the good ol' George Foreman grill and take a pair of kitchen scissors to the chicken, cutting all visible fat off and slicing the breasts smaller and thinner so that they cook faster. I also like to sprinkle various spices and seasonings on the meat before cooking it. I'll set a timer so that I don't have to think too hard about when it will be finished—four and a half to five and a half minutes typically work perfectly.

I like to have enough cooked chicken to last at least two or three days. I'll cut up the rest of the bag of chicken and divide it into freezer bags. Once I finish my cooked chicken, I defrost one of the freezer bags of chicken in the fridge overnight and cook it the following day, which starts the cycle over. Fish can also be frozen, like chicken, but I don't cook as much for later meals. I do not believe it lasts as long, so I eat it right away. You'll quickly find out what works for you and how much you can pre-cook at a time without wasting food. My husband and I go through a lot of chicken!

For your carb sources, you can cook rice ahead of time. If I am making it for my husband and myself, I'll cook about two cups of rice. You can also bake potatoes ahead of time, then either quickly reheat or eat them cold. When I am heading out the door it's very convenient to grab a piece of chicken and small baked potato; this gets me through the next meal while I am out and about.

I also prefer to buy salad mixtures and pre-cut veggies. I realize they are a bit more expensive, but you and I are worth it, and the preparation time it saves will be a treat for you. You can easily add the salad to your cooked chicken, making a nice little meal at any time of the day. Who needs Wendy's or McDonald's to make your salad?

Remember that the more easily available your food is, the better you will eat.

addiction, caffeine should not be cut out straight away. If you feel you may be addicted and would like to use less, start to slowly decrease the amounts you ingest. If you usually drink regular coffee, drink a mixture of half decaf and half regular and then slowly decrease the amount of caffeinated coffee until you are only drinking decaf.

Keep in mind that when you stop caffeine you allow your body to catch up on its lost rest. This takes some time to recover from, since you have been "forcing" yourself with caffeine to produce more energy. For the first few weeks you may find that you are sleeping deeper and for longer periods. This is good! Allow yourself an hour or two of extra sleep per night to regain your normal state and natural energy levels. Be patient with yourself and do not expect it to happen overnight; it may take a few weeks to

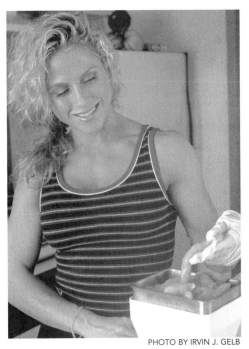

PHOTO BY IRVIN J. GELB

wean yourself completely from your caffeine addiction.

The moral to this story is *drink lots of water* and limit (there's that word again) your intake of soft drinks, tea and coffee.

Alcohol Consumption

Almost everyone asks me if I drink alcohol. I do drink, but I limit the amount, especially if I am preparing for a competition. I have been known to enjoy a glass or two of red or white wine, particularly something like Blackstone Merlot. Any more than two glasses of wine gives me a headache and the munchies—neither of which is fun or good for my body.

I recently came across a "low-carb" wine. How exciting is that? Actually, most wines are fairly low in carbohydrates; from my understanding it depends on the grapes and where they are grown. Data from the U.S. Department of Agriculture states that a five-ounce glass of typical dry red wine contains 102 calories and 2.41 grams of carbohydrates, while typical white wine offers 96 calories and just 1.13 grams of carbs.

Other than wine, I do enjoy a margarita, but I really have to watch those because they have *lots* of carbs and calories—more than I care to know about. I limit my intake to one margarita because I won't feel good if I have two. (Can you tell I really cannot stand to feel bad? It's just not worth it the next day.)

I am *not* recommending that you drink, nor am I saying it is okay to do. It is a very personal decision; I am simply letting you know what I do since I find it is a very common question.

Recipes

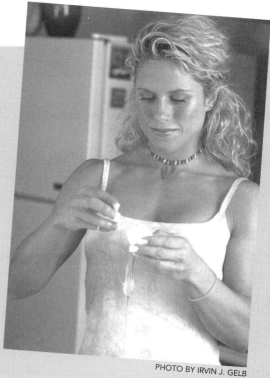

There are so many different ways to make yummy omelets. Be creative and try adding different veggies and meats. Here is one that I enjoy from time to time.

PHOTO BY IRVIN J. GELB

Healthy Omelet
♥ FROM THE KITCHEN OF MONICA BRANT

Ingredients:
5 egg whites
1 oz. cheese (use reduced fat to save calories)
1 cup spinach
½ cup fresh mushrooms and/or onions
2 oz. turkey breast
½ cup cooked brown rice

Directions:
Spray a medium nonstick pan with cooking spray and set heat to medium. Beat the eggs and cook over medium. Flip the omelet as soon as the eggs have set. Sprinkle the other ingredients on the omelet, fold it in half and slide onto plate.

Recipes

Teriyaki Chicken and Rice Bowl
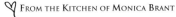 FROM THE KITCHEN OF MONICA BRANT

Ingredients:
5 oz. cooked chicken breast (cooked in my favorite marinade, California Teriyaki
   by Consorzio, but you may use any flavor you enjoy)
1 cup cooked brown or white rice
1 oz. cheddar cheese (use reduced fat to save calories)
2 oz. chopped tomatoes
½ cup shredded lettuce
1 oz. avocado, sliced

Directions:
Cut chicken into bite-sized pieces. Layer chicken and rice in microwave-safe bowl. Heat in microwave. Top with remaining ingredients.

Easy Tacos
FROM THE KITCHEN OF MONICA BRANT

Ingredients:
3-4 oz. chicken breast (raw weight)
2 small (6-inch) corn tortillas
Optional for extra protein: 4 scrambled egg whites
Optional for healthy fats: 1 tbsp. lecithin granules or 1 tbsp. flax seeds
Optional toppings: Green Tabasco sauce, salsa, jalapeños, healthy guacamole (avacados, salsa, seasoning salt, and lime juice mixed together according to taste)

Directions:
Cook chicken on George Foreman or other countertop grill. It will typically cook in four to six minutes, depending on how thick the breast is. Heat corn tortillas either in the microwave or in a hot pan on the stove. If you're heating them on the stove, be sure to turn them a couple times. (Don't burn your fingers!) Slice chicken and layer atop tortillas (add eggs, if using). Add optional items to tacos.

Recipes

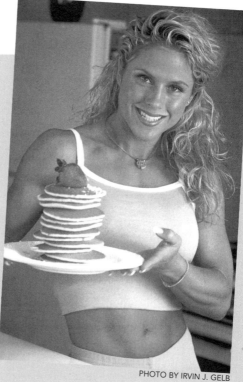

PHOTO BY IRVIN J. GELB

Healthy Pancakes

℘ FROM THE KITCHEN OF MONICA BRANT

Ingredients:
4-5 egg whites
¼ cup cottage cheese
    or 3 ounces extra-firm tofu (use reduced fat to save calories)
½ cup old-fashioned oats
Optional: ½ scoop berry or strawberry flavored protein powder,
    vanilla or almond extract, cinnamon, nutmeg

Directions:
Blend ingredients together in blender. If batter seems too thick, add a very small amount of water or soymilk. Do not over-thin batter. Cook batter like pancakes in heated pan sprayed with cooking spray. Flip when the cake starts to bubble in the pan. Top with Smart Beat butter and/or sugar-free syrup, or just eat plain. These can be made with blueberries, strawberries, or bananas as well, if you are trying to get in some extra calories from carbohydrates. For a very strawberry batch, try using strawberry-flavored oatmeal and a few ripe berries. Yum! The batter will be thin, so add regular old-fashioned oats to thicken.

Recipes

French Toast

♥ FROM THE KITCHEN OF MONICA BRANT

Ingredients:
2-3 slices Vogel brand bread (Vogel bread is made with soy protein and flax seeds)
3 large egg whites, plus 1 yolk, beaten
2 Tbsp. unsweetened soymilk
Optional: dash cinnamon and/or ½ tsp. vanilla
Optional: Smart Beat butter and/or ¼ cup sugar-free syrup

Directions:
Mix the egg and milk (and cinnamon and vanilla, if using) together in a bowl big enough so that the bread will easily soak up the batter. Lightly spray nonstick pan with cooking spray and heat. Dip the bread in the egg mixture and cook on both sides until golden. I like to measure the syrup (starting with a small amount) and dip each bite instead of pouring all of the syrup on the French toast. I use less syrup this way. Remember, even though it says "sugar-free," there are still calories going into your body. Turkey bacon makes a great addition to the French toast for some extra protein.

Tuna Pancake

♥ FROM THE KITCHEN OF MONICA BRANT

Ingredients:
1 small can of water-packed tuna, drained
2 egg whites
½ cup old-fashioned oats

Directions:
Mix ingredients thoroughly in a small bowl. Heat pan sprayed with cooking spray. Shape mixture into a pancake and cook until both sides are lightly browned. Optional: Try adding some mustard or ketchup before indulging.

Recipes

Pizza Snack

ℐ From the Kitchen of Monica Brant

Ingredients:
1 crumpet (in the bread aisle at your local grocery store)
8-10 tofu pepperoni slices
1-2 tbsp. pasta sauce (lowest sugar content available)
1 slice tofu mozzarella cheese
1 slice tofu cheddar cheese

Directions:
Layer all toppings on crumpet and heat in the oven or microwave until the cheese melts. Be careful when taking out and eating, as it will be hot. Of course, this can also be made with real cheese and pepperoni, but doing so will add more fat to the recipe.

Healthy Potato Chips

ℐ From the Kitchen of Monica Brant

Special thanks to Kim Oddo, my nutritionist, for allowing me to use his recipe.

Ingredients:
1 potato, any type
Seasoning, to taste

Directions:
Cut potato into thin rounds and place on microwave-safe plate. Cook in microwave on high for 3-7 minutes, depending how thin you sliced the chips and how powerful your microwave is. You will probably need to do a test run to find out how long they will need to cook in your particular oven. Be careful when removing the plate, as it will be hot. If the chips stick to the plate, take a knife and lift them off. If you are weighing your food for specific amounts, weigh the potatoes before cooking. Season with seasoning salt, sea salt, or any other calorie-free seasoning.

Recipes

Porridge

♈ FROM THE KITCHEN OF MONICA BRANT

Making two servings at once (by doubling the ingredients) makes a convenient and yummy meal later in the day when you need a good carb source. Porridge is great cold, too. I frequently travel with this meal as it lasts well—even through to the second night.

Ingredients:
½ cup old-fashioned oats
4 egg whites (it's easiest if you have these ready to go before starting to cook the oats)
2 packets Splenda or other artificial sweetner
½ scoop vanilla-flavored whey protein powder
Optional: ⅛ cup slivered almonds (measuring is important—fat calories add up quickly)

Directions:
Cook oats as recommended on package. Once oats are boiling, reduce heat to medium and stir the egg whites into the oats. Continue to stir until the eggs cook. You will see them turn white and once the oats are totally finished cooking, the eggs should be done as well. It's about 4-5 minutes total cooking time. At the end of cooking, add the protein powder and Splenda and stir well. Top with almonds if desired.

Ice Cream Sandwich Treats

♈ FROM THE KITCHEN OF MONICA BRANT

You need at least one goodie...here is one of my favorites!

Ingredients:
½ cup Grape-Nuts brand cereal
¼ cup milk chocolate mini-morsels
1-2 cups barely softened low-sugar ice cream (I like Dreyers Grand Light Vanilla, which has half the fat content of regular ice cream)
4-5 graham crackers

Directions:
Mix the cereal and chocolate on a plate and set aside. Spread some ice cream on a graham cracker and place the ice cream side into the mixture on the plate, coating well. Then dip another graham with ice cream into the mixture, coating it well too. Place both halves together, sandwiching the ice cream between the grahams. Make as many as desired, place them inside a freezer bag and freeze. Once they are frozen, the cereal is not so hard and they do not fall apart.

Recipes

Enchilada Lasagna

ℒ FROM THE KITCHEN OF MONICA BRANT

This recipe actually came from a fitness magazine, but I added a few of my own items. I had to include it, since it makes a fairly healthy dish to take for a get-together with friends!

Ingredients:
1 whole chicken
12 corn tortillas
1 package of taco seasoning (medium is my preference)
1 can (15 oz.) of vegetarian refried beans (notice "vegetarian" for less fat)
1 can (10 oz.) of enchilada sauce (medium is my preference)
1 can (10 oz.) of cream of mushroom soup (use reduced fat to save calories)
1 can (4 oz.) of sliced mushrooms
1 ½ cups shredded cheddar cheese (use reduced fat to save calories)

Directions:
Boil the whole chicken for about 35-45 minutes. The chicken will be done when the meat falls off the bones. If the chicken is large you may need to turn it over halfway through the cooking time. Do not overcook the chicken.

Preheat oven to 400 degrees F.

Carefully remove the chicken from pot and separate the meat from the bones and skin. Place the chicken meat in a large bowl and mix in the taco seasoning and enough water to help the seasoning coat the chicken. Add the beans, enchilada sauce, soup and mushrooms and mix well

Spray a 13x9-inch casserole pan with non-stick cooking spray. Spread half of the chicken mixture on the bottom of the pan, add 1/3 of the cheese and top with six tortillas. Repeat the chicken, cheese and tortilla layers, finishing with a layer of cheese on top.

Bake for 30-40 minutes or until the cheese begins to brown and bubble.

Makes 12 servings.

Supplement
Savvy

Supplementation can be one of the most confusing components of the fitness industry. I too become confused at times about what to take, how much to take, and when to take different supplements—specifically, because there are so many variables, different companies, and different opinions on what they do to the body!

However, this makes some sense, too, as our bodies are all very different and some people will experience different effects than others. I know that does not help YOU make up your mind about the what, when, and how much to use, so my best suggestion is to keep to the basics while you are starting your new routine. This will ensure you truly learn what your body is doing with proper nutrition and training prior to adding too many supplements—ones that you may not even need.

Another advantage to keeping your supplementation simple is that your budget will remain in check. Many times I have walked into a nutrition store and ended up leaving with too many things to try. Keeping to the basics will help in the decision-making process, and the next time you need something or want to try something out you will not feel guilty about purchasing things that you have not even used yet. Before starting supple-

mentation, please check with your doctor; some supplements have drug interactions and side effects.

I have prepared a "starter" list of the bare basics of supplements:

- *Multivitamin/multimineral*
- *Vitamin C*
- *Calcium*
- *Glucosamine sulfate*
- *Chondroitin sulfate*
- *Whey protein*
- *Essential fatty acids*

Multivitamin

A **multivitamin** (MV) could be the most important supplement, because the body must be fed a vast array of vital nutrients and minerals to perform at its greatest potential. Allowing deficiencies to occur in our bodies keeps us from performing at our optimum and could cause serious illnesses. Having such copious amounts of unhealthy fast food at our fingertips does not help us either! Much of the food that we consume does not supply our bodies with ample nutrients and minerals to help ensure the presence of essential cofactors necessary for the thousands of metabolic reactions that take place daily in our bodies. Each vitamin and mineral is responsible for certain reactions; if one (or more) is missing, certain functions may not happen as smoothly as possible. Taking a good, reliable MV will help to ensure that you are enabling your body to perform at its peak level.

I prefer to take my MVs in the morning; however, some are designed to be ingested 2-3 times daily to help spread out the dose. I suggest you decide what will be the simplest for you, find a company that

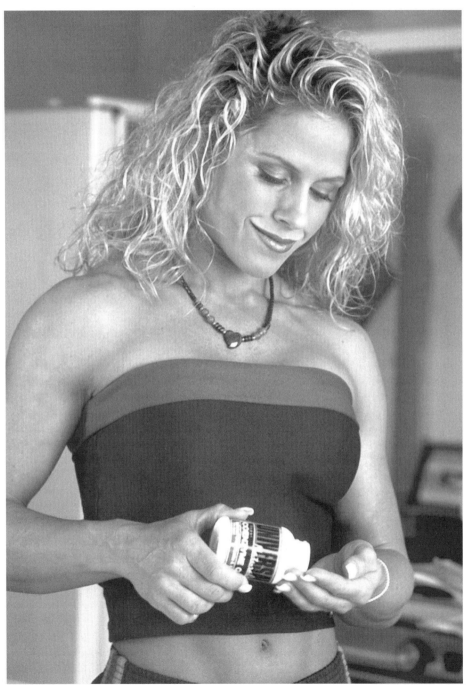

PHOTO BY IRVIN J. GELB

you believe in, and then make a habit of taking the MV.

Keep in mind that MVs are among those supplements that are most likely to have quality problems. Since they contain multiple ingredients, you need to select a MV that has the ingredients you need. You should be confident that it contains what it claims, is free of impurities, and breaks down properly in the body so that the ingredients can be utilized effectively. With so many companies out there, be sure to do some research.

Vitamin C

Another vitamin that is vital to your body is **vitamin C**, also known as ascorbic acid. Vitamin C comes in numerous forms and they are all equally effective. Keep in mind that humans cannot create vitamin C, it is not readily stored, and it is used for a variety of functions—making it necessary to replenish on a daily basis. According to the Linus Pauling Institute, a young, healthy nonsmoker should take at least 400 milligrams of vitamin C every day, "the amount that has been found to fully saturate plasma and circulating cells." The U.S. recommended dietary allowance (RDA) is 75 milligrams a day for women over 19.

Vitamin C has many important roles, according to the Linus Pauling Institute. It is "required for the synthesis of collagen, an important structural component of blood vessels, tendons, ligaments, and bone." Vitamin C affects brain function and mood and is a key in converting fat to energy. "Recent research also suggests that vitamin C...may have implications for blood cholesterol levels.

"Vitamin C is also a highly effective antioxidant. Even in small amounts vitamin C can protect indispensable molecules in the body, such as proteins, lipids (fats), carbohydrates, and nucleic acids (DNA and RNA) from damage by free radicals and reactive oxygen species that can be generated during normal metabolism as well as through exposure to toxins and pollutants (e.g., smoking)."

Speaking of smoking, hopefully I do not have to remind any of you that smoking is horribly dangerous to your body. I find it hard to accept that anyone who trains and works hard to eat properly can also enjoy smoking—disregarding the long- and short-term effects it has on one's body! Not only are you severely damaging *your* body, but you are also damaging your loved ones and your pets. Please, if not for yourself, consider others if you are a smoker!

Anyway, back to vitamin C: I increase my intake when traveling and working at conventions where I interact with thousands of people. Studies have demonstrated that large doses of vitamin C (2 grams) have been found to decrease the duration and severity of the common cold.

Calcium

Next on the starter supplement list is **calcium**, which is the most abundant mineral in the body and is essential for many important functions. Even though it can be obtained by eating leafy green veggies and dairy products, many people still do not get the recommended daily amounts. I am quite positive that I do not get enough from the foods I eat, since I limit my dairy and I can only eat leafy green veggies so many times a day.

Calcium is most noted for providing for healthy bones and teeth. It also helps regulate many important functions of the heart, cellular membranes, and kidneys. Chronic calcium deficiencies contribute to osteoporosis, a major threat to a healthy body. I typically consume 1,000 milligrams per day.

Glucosamine sulfate & Chondroitin sulfate

Because of our fast-paced lives and intense exercise programs, I feel that our joints and connective tissue need to be pampered some, too! Also on the starter list are the building blocks of healthy joints and tissue: **glucosamine sulfate** and **chondroitin sulfate**. These products can help repair damaged joints and aid in tissue repair. If you have bad knees, elbows, or wrists, chances are these products may help you. I use a product that is made only with glucosamine and chondroitin, as opposed to one that has other vitamins as well.

Whey protein & Essential fatty acids

Rounding out my list are **whey protein** and **essential fatty acids**, which I discussed in the protein and fat sections, respectively.

One more point regarding whey: If you are lactose intolerant and are concerned about using a whey protein powder, look for a whey product that says "lactose free" on the label. Most "isolate" types of whey use a filtering technique that will remove virtually all lactose.

Advanced Supplementaton

If you are training seriously and are looking toward the next level of supplementation, you might consider **glutamine**. Glutamine is a nonessential amino acid. Nonessential does not mean "unimportant;" it just means that the body can produce it. (Just to remind you, amino acids are the building blocks of proteins and muscle tissue. All physiological processes relating to sport—energy, recovery, muscle gain/strength, and fat loss—as well as brain and mood functions are linked to amino acids.)

Even though our body is able to produce glutamine under normal conditions, in times of high stress, glutamine reserves become depleted and need to be replenished. High stress can be caused by intense activities, work, sickness, and emotional imbalances.

I typically take glutamine powder mixed in water immediately after training, sprinting, and before bedtime to ensure I am properly "glutamined." In my opinion, glutamine's combination of positive benefits and lack of side effects makes it a product almost everyone can use with confidence!

The last item you may be interested in is a **fat burner** supplement. If you are interested in taking a fat burner, you should check with your doctor, as some people have adverse reactions to them. My view on fat burners in general is that they should NOT be taken without proper supervision and should NOT be used unless a strict nutrition plan and training routine is being followed. If you have consulted a doctor and are following a regulated plan, supplementing your efforts with a fat burner is, in my opinion, okay. I recommend starting with only one capsule or tablet in the morning before breakfast to see how your body will react. Try this for one week and if all goes well, add a second capsule in the early afternoon for one week. If that is also acceptable for your body, try taking two capsules in the morning and one in the afternoon.

Do not stay on fat burners for more than eight weeks from start to finish. I also recommend weaning the fat burner out of your system gradually to help your body to ease back into its normal rhythm of fat reduction. Keep in mind that your appetite might increase without the aid of fat burners and you may need a bit more discipline!

Unfortunately, some people become addicted to fat burners and think they cannot stay fit or lean without them. If you become dependent, I suggest easing them out of your system gently. Getting extra sleep, increasing water intake, and adding a few extra interval minutes to your cardio sessions will help keep your metabolism moving. You must allow your body to function on its own—without stimulants—from time to time!

Almost all the products I mentioned above provide some sort of sickness prevention. Even though you may be supplying your body with the necessary supplements for a healthy body, you may still come down with the common cold or worse. It would seem that remaining healthy is relatively easy if you are able to eat, drink, exercise, and rest appropriately; however, our busy lifestyles do not leave much room for extra rest or time to eat properly every day, which leaves room for sickness to creep in!

I am sure it is the same for you: Getting sick is one of my biggest irritations! Even though I do not fall sick regularly, the times that I do are never convenient. To speed recovery, I take extra care to drink plenty of water, increase my vitamin C intake, and eat natural foods that will provide me with good nutrition.

Rest is definitely important to recovery and I often cut back on my training and cardio sessions depending on the degree of sickness. You will have to gauge your body's needs and take the necessary steps to recover. Sometimes pushing yourself will only make it worse and then you will be out even longer! Do not be afraid to take the day off and give yourself some needed rest.

How to Get and Stay
MOTIVATED

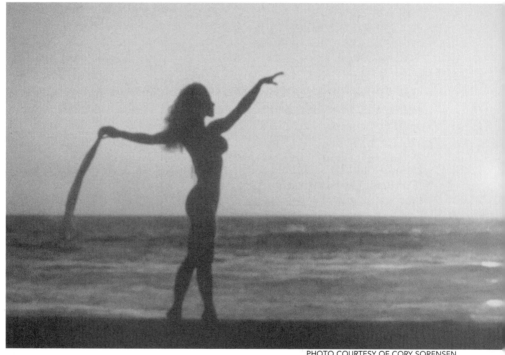

PHOTO COURTESY OF CORY SORENSEN

Nothing is more
powerful
than habit.

—Ovid

Habit is
overcome
by habit.

—Thomas a Kempis

I decided that the best way to start this chapter would be to answer the most popular question that is asked of me. Within the last two years or so, friends, fans, and family wonder how I stay motivated to remain in this industry for so long, since for the past decade I have been constantly competing, training, traveling (sometimes weekly), and eating to remain as fit as possible. After all, no one wants to see an out-of-shape fitness/figure competitor giving a seminar!

That said, I do believe this could be the most important chapter for many of you. So, I will do my absolute best to express myself—my thoughts and feelings—and hopefully I will impart courage, inspiration, and resolution to you! My goal is to help you become the person you want to be or to make the changes you need to make.

With this in mind, I definitely believe that a mixture of things motivate me. Sometimes motivation comes in the form of a desire to accomplish a personal goal, while other times the motivation is spiri-

tual, financial, friends and family, and of course, fans. Many of the e-mails and letters I receive are very inspirational—some even bring tears to my eyes!

Before we delve any further, let's take a look at the word "motivation" and see what it really implies. (I have a fascination with looking up words in the dictionary—sometimes I have to know exactly what a definition is before I can totally understand a concept. I even have the website *www.dictionary.com* bookmarked for convenience on my computer!)

> "Motivation: *n:* the psychological feature that arouses an organism to action toward a desired goal; the reason for the action; that which gives purpose and direction to behavior..."

The first thing I noticed in the definition above is the word "psychological" (okay, I looked up *psychological* too: "arising from the mind or emotions"). So, motivation arouses an organism (*you* and *me*) to action toward a desired *goal*! You see right away that motivation is psychological and has to come from within *yourself* first. I feel that my own willpower is definitely one of the biggest motivating factors in my life. For example, if I decide to do something, I will be disciplined and determined, striving to be the best I can be for that particular goal.

Now let's look at the rest of that definition...something about goals. Goals—yes, I have to have goals in order to have motivation! I think this may be the reason many people lack motivation. I believe motivation is definitely driven by both short- and long-term goals, so let's take a closer look at making, meeting, and exceeding your goals.

Goal
Setting

Goals have to be intertwined in our lives for our satisfaction and happiness. When people lack goal-setting skills, they may find themselves depressed and dragging through life, barely able to get through normal everyday tasks.

To really begin at square one, try giving yourself simple tasks to do—tasks that you know you will be able to achieve and feel good about. I think it is important to have successes each day, even if they are small. Small successes will give you confidence to ask more of yourself, thus achieving larger goals and ultimately living a much happier life.

One of the best ways I have found to live out my dreams and goals is by writing them down. Even if they are only short-term, I find it fun to cross out goals on the "to do" list as I accomplish them each day. (This also helps keep me organized and productive.) My day planner is filled with items for the day such as:

7:00 am—Wake up, drink a
    protein shake
7:45 am—45-60 minute run outside
8:45 am—Clean up, eat breakfast
10:00 am—Start working in the office
12:30 pm—Eat lunch
12:45 pm—Back to office
4:00 pm—Eat again; run errands
    (post office, photo lab, tan, nails)
7:00 pm—Train
8:00pm—Eat dinner, CALL MOM!

I have a better chance of successfully meeting my short-term goals when I plan out my entire day. As I eat or run errands, I can cross those off my list and feel like I accomplished something. Even if it was a small task, the bottom line is I made it happen!

Successfully meeting short-term goals helps instill confidence in your ability to also meet long-term goals. Do not be afraid to write down your thoughts and dreams, even if they seem far-fetched! Keep a notebook and jot down your ideas whenever you have them. I actually keep mine with my notebook that I use for phone calls and notes concerning jobs and plans. This way I can look back at the end of the year, review all the events, and make sure I did not forget a specific idea.

Another step to setting personal goals is to really get to know yourself. Learn what you like and what makes you "tick;" this will help you establish your goals and ultimately follow your dreams. Knowing who you really are, what you really enjoy, and what you are capable of will help you set realistic goals for yourself.

One of the ways you can get to know yourself is to spend some time in silence. For example, instead of turning on the morning news when you first wake up, listen to your mind and heart and see how you are feeling that day. We are constantly asking others how they are feeling; why not find out how you are feeling too?

My personal favorite and most effective method of getting inside myself is to read some scripture and talk to God. Taking the time to say good morning to God with prayer when I am preparing my food for the day helps me to ground myself and feel joyful, which usually leads to a very productive day.

I figure God made me, so He should be fully capable of directing my path and helping me to prioritize my day fluidly! Also, giving thanks for his blessings seems to help with motivation tremendously. Sometimes when I think I lack motivation or direction, what I am really lacking is some good ol' quiet time with my Creator.

I have even noticed that the times when I am craving goodies or snacks and I reach for some food to satiate my tummy, what is really happening is my *spirit* is lacking attention! I have always felt that I need a good balance between nutritional, spiritual, physical, and emotional needs. I realize that when I do not take as much time for my inside (nutritional, spiritual, and emotional) needs, my outside suffers! I find this truly amazing!

Visualize

Visualization is a great tool to help you accomplish your now-written-down goals. Years ago, when I was preparing for my fitness competitions, I would visualize my routine while I did cardio. Since I was concentrating on my visualization and not the time, the minutes ticked by quickly. I burned fat and clearly thought through each and every move in my routine, which resulted in more fluid transitions and movements the next day at practice!

In order to get the visualization process going for you, ask yourself the following questions: What is my ultimate dream? What visual image will I work toward? Do I want to be smaller? More fit? Stronger? More muscular? (One of my biggest dreams is to become a taller me.

Ha! Too bad that can't happen with visualization!)

Remember that a dream is a vision of the future. So dream of yourself in the future as the hottest thing alive! Visualize yourself in the best shape possible—wearing that cute little black dress to the company party or the tight jeans you just saw in one of your favorite stores. It can happen! All you have to do is make a conscious decision about your goals so that you can then start to visualize making them happen.

If you've had the same body structure for most of your life, you might have a hard time visualizing yourself differently. This is where finding a role model could come in handy. Finding someone you can relate to (even if it is only in hair color) might help you focus your visualization of yourself.

Throughout my years in this industry I have been privileged to view many photos from ladies who have taken "before and after" shots. I always ask them if they ever dreamed they could look as good as they do in the "after" shots. They usually say they had no idea what their body looked like under that layer of fat. But they dreamed a dream, worked on their goals, and, lo and behold, look what they had under that layer!

I believe that our Heavenly Father gave each of us a lifetime project—our bodies. He calls them our temples, which is pretty serious stuff. I believe God expects us to take care of this project He has blessed us with. In fact, I challenge you to make your project as healthy as possible!

Can you believe you are the only one who can make it happen? How neat is it to think that no one else can do this for you? You are in total control of how your project will turn out!

Recently I have been studying *The Testimony of the Evangelists* by Dr. Simon Greenleaf (1783-1853). In case you are unfamiliar with Dr. Greenleaf, he was one of the principle founders of Harvard Law School.

You will have to read it sometime if you are interested in his conclusion about the evangelists, the Gospels, and the resurrection of Jesus Christ.

Dr. Greenleaf made a statement that I feel can be applied to our pursuit of a healthy project or "temple":

"It should be pursued as in the presence of God, and under the solemn sanctions created by a lively sense of his omniscience, and of our accountability to Him for the right use of the faculties which He has bestowed."

In other words, we are accountable to our Creator with our bodies and what we do with and to them! Get busy, girl!

The Follow-Through: Habits

The follow-through is the toughest part. It is easy to say, "Yes, I am going to do this and yes, I *can!*" The follow-through has to be thought about as a continual part of life, something that will never change, no matter how old you are.

I try to keep it on the same level as brushing my teeth. I know that if I do not brush and floss, my teeth will eventually rot and fall out. *Yuck!* So why would it be any different for our bodies? Why not show the same discipline for our physiques?

Parents teach children at a very young age about brushing their teeth. I can still remember my dad telling me that I have to keep my "little white doggies" clean. I think if parents spent the time teaching children to eat healthy in the young stages of life they might grow up with a different attitude about food. My mom cooked tasty meals and she never (to my knowledge) worried about us eating too much fat or carbs. However, I was *very* athletic growing up and I am quite positive that any extra calories were quickly burned. I believe that children should be allowed the occasional treat now and then, but junk food shouldn't be readily available at all times. Also, children need to learn to exercise— not just watch TV and play video games. Imagine the difference it could make in a child's future if he or she was taught to exercise regularly. Think about it: What we are taught in childhood, will be practiced in adulthood. Why not learn about healthy eating and appropriate exercise early on in life?

Following through really comes down to breaking old habits and establishing new, healthier habits. Let's see, just for fun, what the dictionary says about habits.

"Habit: n: a thing done often and hence easily; a usual way of doing; an addiction."

If we can alter our habits to fit our needs, our goals will become easier to attain. Like anything, the more you practice, the easier something becomes. This is also true when it comes to eating and exercising.

What habits do you have that keep you from having that dream physique? Do you even realize what habits are keeping you back? Maybe it is that late-night habit of eating chips and watching some TV to fall asleep. This seems to be fairly common. If I cannot fall asleep, I will grab the Bible and read some scriptures, which typicaly brings sleep fast. Ha! At least I am falling asleep to something that brings peace to my soul and spirit.

The idea is to figure out which habits are keeping you from success—and then ease out of them. Like anything addictive, I suggest cutting back slowly or replacing your bad habit with something else. If you're talking about late-night snacks, consider having cucumbers prior to bedtime for something crunchy and filling.

To get to know your bad habits, try writing them down so you accept them for what they are and for the damage they can do. I say "accept," because I don't think we can change bad habits if we don't really accept them as bad habits. If you're unsure of your bad habits, ask a loved one who knows you best. I am sure they will know!

Next to your bad habits, counter with a good habit! This way you have a rule to go by. Write down your bad habits in black and your good habits in your favorite color.

In summary, here's how you can begin the process of meeting and exceeding your fitness goals:

1. Learn about yourself
2. Figure out your goals and write them down
3. Visualize what you will become
4. Make a decision
5. Challenge yourself to follow through
6. Follow through and change (For me, I ask God to help me follow through)

What About Willpower?

"What about willpower?" you ask. Willpower is definitely a good thing to have, and one needs a lot of it to succeed. Of course it will be different for everyone, since we all have different strengths. Breaking bad habits takes a lot of willpower.

Just look at the words *will* and *power*—what do they tell you? Your dedication (will) has to be powerful.

When was the last time you were powerful in the way you trained? When was the last time you were powerful in your eating plan for the entire week (or month)? Why not challenge yourself now to be powerful in your decisions?

I realize it is not easy to be disciplined and focused each day. For me it's hardest when I am tired or run down from traveling the world. Those are the days that I have to dig deep and pull out the willpower. Unfortunately, no one can do this part for you. No one can make you put the best food choices in your mouth or pick you up and carry you to the gym. (Wouldn't that be nice though?) These are things we (including me) have to make choices about every day.

Motivation
From
Others

Back to the original topic of this chapter—motivation. Motivation comes from different sources, and not each source will work for all occasions. For example, if I decide to make a goal of competing again I will first talk it over with my husband to make sure he is in agreement with me. (FYI, if you have a partner, it is important that he is supportive of what you want to do—whether it be competing or just simply joining a gym to get in better shape.) Together, we figure out if the competition is feasible with what is going on in our lives at the time.

My husband is a main source of motivation for me. At the time of writing this book we have only been married for one year—and I have no idea how I survived for so long without his support! I had to make decisions and plans on my own for so many years. If you have a partner, I encourage you to get him involved in your dreams and ask him to help you. Men typically enjoy knowing they can help—maybe your husband or boyfriend would be a big source of motivation for you, too. But keep in mind that if you ask for his help in supporting you and helping you to eat better (for example), then do not be frustrated when he pulls that piece of bread out of your mouth!

My next motivational step is to dig up old contest photos that showcase my physique in both the best shape and the worst. Viewing my past photos helps me

to be realistic in my thoughts about preparing for the show. They help me visualize what I need to do in order to compete at the level I need to be. Photos are a great source of motivation for me! They remind me of where I was and where I want to be again.

Other than my husband, photos, and willpower, my motivation can also come from friends and fans! Many times I have received the nicest e-mails or letters from fans around the world who share their stories of success and how I have been a source of inspiration for them. I am amazed every time I read these—amazed that I could be that big of an influence on someone's life. I am honored with such sincere stories; these stories in turn give me that extra boost for my day and for my own personal goals.

I have collected many wonderful letters along the way and I wanted to share a few with you. I am hoping that you will find some encouragement in the letters, and know that you, too, can make the changes you would like to make for yourself.

"my true description of a hero"

Aside from a flawless physique and stunning beauty, Monica is one of the most inspiring and motivational figures in my life. As an overweight little girl I used to spend hours on end cutting out her photos from any magazine I could find her in. I would study the advice she gave readers and dream to build a masterpiece like hers. Gathering the information she gave out and following in her footsteps, I progressed from an over-weight teenager to a seasoned competitor and fitness model with Monica as my motivation. Despite her busy schedule and plethora of activities, she never fails to take the time to help me develop into my own personal best. She is my true description of a hero. Her fervor for life and relationship with God has motivated me time and time again and encouraged me both as an athlete and a woman of God.

Priscilla Tuft

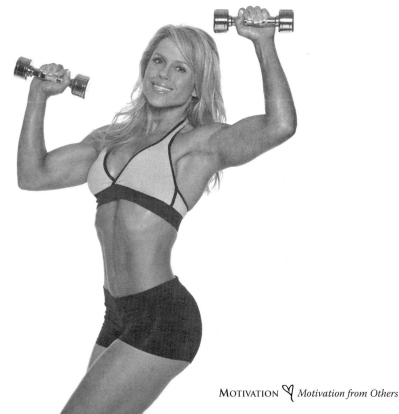

"wealth of fitness information"

Monica possesses the rare and priceless gift of seeing the potential in everyone she meets and then encouraging them to pursue the excellence inside them.

However, her one-of-a-kind gifting doesn't stop there.

Monica is a genuine person who will inspire, encourage, motivate and promote another person's success without showing jealousy, intimidation, or having any expectations of being given something back in return for her goodwill.

Monica truly desires that everyone reach their full potential physically, mentally, emotionally, and spiritually, as she shamelessly references her faith in God.

For me, as an indie Christian singer/songwriter, she is a breath of fresh air when I've been stagnant, a hand up when I've fallen, and new inspiration when I've given up.

She is a wealth of fitness information, but isn't arrogant. For me, she is the best source of fitness know-how, but she doesn't display an air of superiority.

All these things that she is, professionally and personally, make her what she is summed up to be: She is loved!

Eva Sandiford

"muscles ARE sexy"

When I first started lifting as a teenager, I purchased a *Muscle & Fitness* magazine and there inside was Monica Brant. I was immediately inspired by her physique and how beautiful she looked. My thoughts were: "Muscles ARE sexy on women!" Monica has always been my absolute favorite!

When I turned 19, I got married and moved to the U.S. A few years went by and after having a child at the age of 23, I had gained 55 pounds, going from 140 pounds up to 195 pounds. By the time my daughter turned 20 months old, I had become unhealthy and my body fat had gone up to 32% at 142 pounds.

When I heard my husband say to me, "Do you want me to paint those on you?" referring to my size 12 jeans, I knew it was time to start lifting again! That's when I decided to make a lifestyle change, set myself goals, and have a role model. Who better than Monica Brant? I posted an 8" x 10" picture where I could see it every day as a reminder of how good I could look if I put in time and effort to achieve my goals.

Today I'm a fit and healthy mommy and wife! In just 12 weeks of hard work and dedication I was able to bring my body fat down from 32% to 18.8%. I lost 18 pounds of fat and gained nine pounds of muscle. I now wear a size six! I'm in the best shape of my life and look forward to continuing this new lifestyle.

Thanks, Monica, for your hard work and dedication to your fans. You are God's blessing to many of us! You've inspired me and I hope my letter will do the same.

Sincerely yours,

Carole Ingram

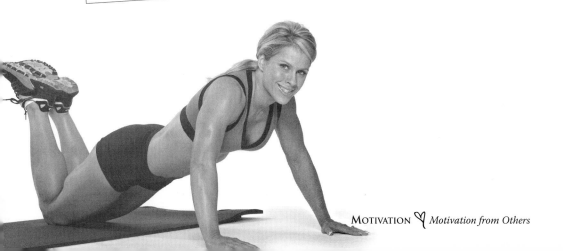

"positive influence was a catalyst"

At the milestone of age 40, I looked back and realized that every once in a while someone steps into your life and somehow changes your direction. Monica Brant is one of those individuals.

The 2002 BodyRock/Monica Brant Fitness Classic was my first experience of fitness competition. I was nervous and at the same time excited to meet Monica Brant, one of the women I admired on the covers of fitness magazines for years. At first I was a little star struck; she was absolutely stunning and even more beautiful in person. Besides her sheer physical beauty, I was equally impressed to learn Monica was genuinely selfless and kind. She was totally involved and attentive with all of us girls backstage. I appreciated the way she stuck right by her competitors for the entire day and helped us with everything from applying tanning oil to hair and makeup.

Monica Brant was my first major role model of how a fitness professional should conduct themselves. Her positive influence was a catalyst for some of my future career choices.

Motivated to move up the competitive fitness ladder, I won first place at the 2003 NPC National Fitness Championships (middle height class). Fitness was a great experience, but I am now taking some time off from the physical stress of competitive Fitness to focus on competing in Pro Figure. Now into my second season of professional competition, I am certain to miss the performance aspect of Fitness, but I am enjoying my training for Figure. I am also involved in some very exciting career opportunities, such as a fitness DVD and personal website.

Speaking of careers, another impressive and influential quality Monica possesses is her business savvy. I can tell that not only does she love what she is doing, but it is a business for her. This too influenced my future in Fitness. I remember visiting Monica's website over and over to stay motivated and to study her physique, hoping that someday I could look like her. I enjoyed reading and learning from all of her valuable information about training, nutrition, and expert beauty tips. She was a powerful mentor for me with my own fitness business.

After seeing Monica grace the covers of countless magazines and many of the pages in between, one of my dreams was to one day see myself in a magazine and when that finally happened I was thrilled. It has been an exciting ride so far and I will never forget my humble beginnings nor the people who have helped positively changed my life, especially Monica Brant.

Monica Brant, I thank you for all of your goodness. You probably don't realize how much you have changed my life. Your inspiration has helped shape the wonderful world I'm enjoying today!

I'm forever grateful,

Lydia Haskell
IFBB Fitness & Figure Pro

"an elegance that comes from deep within"

How did I become inspired by Monica Brant? First, I think it was a certain inner beauty that showed through! I had received an *Oxygen* magazine that had pictures of the 2004 figure competition in Las Vegas, and as I looked at all of the pictures, there was Monica's. She seemed to possess an elegance that comes from deep within, and I could see and feel this from her picture. Her makeup did not look over-done and there was a confidence that she really knew who she was…and was very proud of that.

After going to her website and then e-mailing her, I got even more of that honesty from her. I went to a few more websites that had other pictures of her competing. There was just something that I had to have. I wanted to put her in my right-hand pocket and have her train me and take her everywhere with me…

What inspired me, too, was that I had read an article that stated that she was a Christian and that in her field of work, she takes that belief with her. She bases her life around God and a determination to succeed.

Having been a fan of the figure competitors and dreaming of one day achieving a body like Monica's, I set my hopes and dreams on my upcoming wedding. With Monica being a fan to me and cheering me on, wishing me luck with the upcoming wedding, I got the incentive to push even harder. Then she e-mailed me about her t-shirts and I received both of them and one was autographed! I found that kept me going even more.

Today, I say a prayer every morning to God to help me achieve my goals and my dreams. Knowing that Monica is rooting for me and sending little spiritual messages through the grapevine keeps me going.

(continued on page 104)

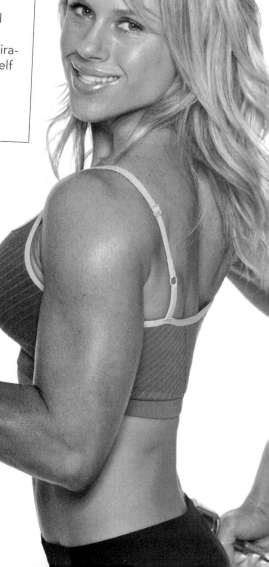

With a healthy diet and exercise I have lost approximately 15 pounds. The best part of this is that I am 41 years old and I also have a six-year-old...Plus, I have two part-time jobs. So finding the time to exercise was not an easy accomplishment. I could come up with any reason to not exercise. Now with the help of Monica's pictures, I put my exercise and my health first. I am much stronger and happier when I say I need to do this for me.

Anyone that really and truly, deeply and honestly wants something passionately enough, can and will have what is desired, but getting into action is the first step. So, thank you, Monica, for being my inspiration and for telling me that I inspire you. That in itself is motivation for me.

Teri Wyekoff-Hardwick

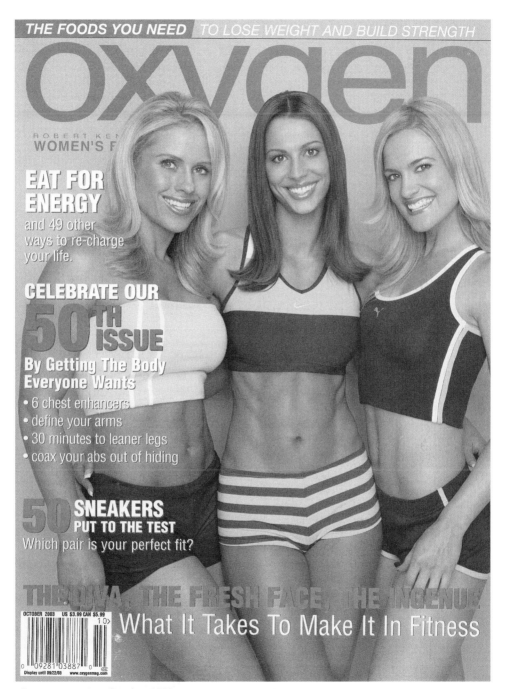

THE FOODS YOU NEED TO LOSE WEIGHT AND BUILD STRENGTH

OXygen

ROBERT KEN
WOMEN'S F

EAT FOR ENERGY
and 49 other ways to re-charge your life.

CELEBRATE OUR
50TH ISSUE

By Getting The Body Everyone Wants
- 6 chest enhancers
- define your arms
- 30 minutes to leaner legs
- coax your abs out of hiding

50 SNEAKERS
PUT TO THE TEST
Which pair is your perfect fit?

THE DIVA, THE FRESH FACE, THE INGENUE

What It Takes To Make It In Fitness

OCTOBER 2003   US $3.99 CAN $5.99
10>
0 09281 03887 6
Display until 09/22/03   www.oxygenmag.com

Oxygen magazine, October 2003. Used with permission.

Ask Monica:
Questions
Answers

How strict do I really have to be to get in amazing shape like the women I see competing in Fitness?

Sadly, I have found many believe the ultimate dream is to achieve the "fitness competitor" extreme lean-body look, but unless your goal is to step on stage, it is very unrealistic to strive for that extremely low level of body fat.

If that is the leanness you are expecting, you may never be completely happy with yourself, and you'll miss out on the joy you can have being contented with a normal, healthy body.

The levels of fat that a competitor has for stage are for the stage only. It's not realistic to maintain such a level for more than a couple days. Competitors flush water so that their bodies are almost in a dehydrated state come stage time. This is definitely not convenient to a normal day in the life of a non-competitor.

It is extremely challenging to become that lean (5-8% body fat) and it takes many weeks and sometimes months to look like that for one or two days. If this is your view of what YOUR body needs to look like, please listen and trust when I say this is NOT the look you should want, unless of course your desire is to compete, and that is another story for another book!

I believe it is very important to have a realistic mental picture of the shape you CAN be. One that, with hard work and dedication, you can achieve and LOVE! You need to love the way you look and feel—if you, do you will radiate health and vitality to all that are near you, and you will find yourself answering all sorts of questions regarding what you are up to. Everyone will think you are on a magic pill! At least they are hoping that you are, and that you will share your information with them!

ASK MONICA: Questions & ANSWERS

What can be done to help with my posture? I find myself slouching and hunching forward a lot. Are there any exercises that could help me? I do not want to be a hunched-over elderly lady!

I understand your pain—when I was growing up I can remember my mom correcting my posture and telling me to hold in my stomach and stand up straight. I can still remember a few photos taken when I was young, with my belly sticking out and my lower back arched. I have a feeling that had my mom not been so persistent with me, I would have ended up with a serious back problem. At any rate, I believe you can definitely change your posture at any age.

Regarding exercise, I suggest doing Pilates (a method of physical and mental exercise involving stretching and breathing that focuses on strengthening the abdominal core) two to three times weekly, as your core may lack strength. Also, deep tissue massage can be effective for loosening tight muscles, which could be the cause of your posture problems.

One of the things I notice in myself is that I have very poor eyesight, and many times I find myself hunched forward to read the computer screen, causing my posture to suffer. To avoid this I use a large font and bold letters when typing so that I can sit back in the seat and keep my shoulders back. Yes, I am wearing contacts, too! You might also have your eyes checked to ensure proper vision.

Try jotting a few notes for yourself, saying "Perfect Posture, Girl" and tape them to your car, mirror, computer, fridge…anywhere you will see them on a regular basis to help remind yourself to straighten up.

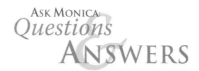

Should I weigh myself on a scale and if so, how often?

I am not one to weigh myself except for a very few select times per year. Fortunately, I have never purchased a scale to keep at home, and most of the time when I consider weighing myself at the scale in the gym, there's already a guy on it! HA!

In my opinion, weighing yourself can be addictive and mentally unhealthy because most of us are NEVER happy with what we weigh. We always think we should weigh less (or more, for some of you lucky "fast metabolism" ladies).

There are many variables regarding weight, such as hormones, water retention, travel schedules, eating, sleeping, health issues, and so on. Weighing yourself one day will only cause you to be curious the next, and then it just seems to get into a vicious cycle of constantly worrying about weight.

I have always based my weight on how my clothes are fitting. If they are feeling too tight, then I do not need a scale to tell me that I'm too heavy.

If you have to weigh yourself, try not to do it every day. Instead, do it maybe once a week or every 10 days. Also, weigh yourself at the same time of day before your training and cardio. Use the same scale so that you have an accurate record.

I prefer to have my body fat levels tested instead of stepping on a scale. I do this as I am preparing for competitions, once a week on Sunday mornings before training legs. I have my nutritionist pinch me, and we keep track of my progress each week. This does help me stay focused!

Can you give me some tips on choosing a gym?

Choosing where you will train will definitely help you with the "getting to the gym" problem. Convenience is key with how busy we all are in this day and age. If you're new to the area, I suggest making a list of the gyms closest to you and then going to each one of them and "interviewing" them. Pay attention to how the staff greets you and how educated they seem to be. If you are new to training and need some assistance, find out if they are able to assist you in the gym and what their credentials are. You will want to feel comfortable in your new home! Also, ask about child care if you will need it and be sure to check out the ladies room. See how clean it is and what amenities are offered.

Make a checklist of the things that are important to you, and then take some time at each gym to find the one that suits you best. After you decide on one or two gyms you think might work, ask if you can have a week pass to try it out. This request should not be an issue with the gym. If it is, I would move on to the next gym!

I truly believe that you will find it very difficult to get to a gym that is not convenient at least to your home or work. Do not fool yourself into believing that you won't mind driving more than 15-20 minutes to the gym—unless of course you live in the country and that's the location of your nearest gym. Making time for the gym has to be easy as possible so that you do not put it off.

As you choose your gym, don't forget about another important aspect of your training—scheduling. I recommend writing your weekly training schedule into your day planner. Scheduling training into your day/week will help you keep track of what you have already trained, what is to come, and help you stay focused. Be sure to schedule your week realistically. There's no need to write down something you know you will not be able to do! If you find you are able to fulfill your realistic schedule, then think about adding another 10-15 minutes after each session for some good stretching.

ASK MONICA:
Questions &
ANSWERS

What do I do when I'm asked to go to a favorite restaurant where I'm sure to blow my diet? What if you live with someone who does not eat the same way that you do?

For me it would definitely depend on where I am in my contest year. If I am close to a competition, I might have to ask for a rain check, unless there is some urgency. (Perhaps a friend needs some emotional support—then I would definitely go.) If I am just maintaining my condition and not near a contest, I would go and enjoy a good dinner with my friend.

Yes, that means eating the calamari and having that glass of wine, though we would probably share the dessert. You can do this too and not feel guilty. The only thing you will want to do for sure is make your other meals very healthy both during the day before dinner and the day after dinner. This will help balance out the meal that was not on your program. You do not have to give up all good-tasting meals for the rest of your life. It is all about moderation.

To answer the second part of your question, if you live with someone who has a hard time accepting what you're trying to do with your physique, try sitting him or her down and explaining exactly what it is that you are hoping to achieve and why.

Maybe you have a female roommate who could use a healthier eating routine. Ask her to join you in your quest for a better physique. Maybe you could end up being her motivation! I do believe we are all motivating factors to the people in our surroundings.

You may not even know the impact you have already made on someone's life. I call it the domino effect. We all have it going on, just at different levels.

Fortunately the only female roommate I had was a very close friend who was also involved in Fitness. She and I had a great time buying food for each other. We would share our healthy foods and replace what we ate. (Okay, we'd also share the unhealthy foods. HA!)

I enjoy looking my best at the gym, but am frustrated by how expensive the clothing is! How do you clean your clothes to extend the wear of them and keep them looking new?

I, too, find that workout wear is very expensive, especially if you buy the brands that use a good quality, thick material with patterns, and "dance pants!" I think the best way to keep these expensive items fresh and bright is to wash them separately with other similar clothing, such as other workout wear, undergarments, cute t-shirts, etc. Definitely do not wash them with jeans or anything that will be "hard" on them. DO wash and rinse them in COLD (even my light colors) and set the machine to the delicate cycle. Adding color-safe bleach, like Clorox 2, to the wash will help with colors as well!

Also, I never dry any of my workout wear in the dryer. I know it takes more time, but I hang dry them every time on a collapsible drying rack. You can find smooth wooden or metal ones at most discount retail stores and they fold up to fit easily in your closet.

Something of interest is a new laundry detergent that is just hitting the market called WIN High Performance Sport Detergent. In fact, it is the new official detergent of Olympic athletes! It is designed to remove embedded sweat and odors from workout clothing. I assume that having cleaner clothes will extend the wear of them too! Check out this revolutionary product on the web at www.winproductsinc.com.

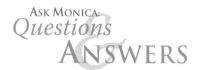

I am so confused. What should I drink or eat POST-workout? Please help!

This is a great question! You are correct; post-workout recovery nutrition is very important! There are many different opinions floating around in the fitness industry today, but the main thing to remember is to just get something in!

Two very valuable supplements, glutamine and branched chain amino acids, are probably your number one and two items to take for muscle recovery and recuperation. I like to carry them to the gym with me and mix them immediately after training/cardio—that way I do not leave the gym without taking them!

Next on the agenda for post-workout recovery should be a small meal of lean protein and a simple carbohydrate or slightly higher glycemic carb such as a potato.

Fast-releasing protein shakes (whey isolate) are very good for this as well, since they are basically predigested and will enter your bloodstream quickly, making it to your muscles in a flash.

Regardless of whether you eat a meal or drink a shake, for optimal results, try not to allow more than 30-45 minutes to go by without some nutrition—this is your best window for rapid recovery.

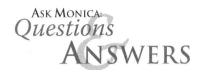

What is your feeling about breast implants?

I hope this small section of the book does not offend anyone, but this has been a major question that many ladies have asked me over the years, and I feel it is appropriate to address the issue.

First, please let me say that I do not believe that a woman's chest makes her who she is. I know many women who are beautiful and confident with breasts of all sizes, enhanced or not.

Second, remember that a woman's breast is made up of fatty tissue and glands. It is almost guaranteed that 95 percent of women are going to lose breast size as they start to train, eat healthy, and lose body fat. Unfortunately there is NOTHING you can do about it. Of course, training chest will strengthen your chest muscles and keep your posture nice, but it will not build your breast tissue (cup size). For those of you hoping to increase your breast size and decrease your body fat, I am afraid the only route you can go is surgery. Please let me also clarify that I have always encouraged women to only go under the knife if it is something THEY want, not at their husband's, friends', or boyfriend's request. There should be no regrets!

Back in October of 1993, after dieting for a couple shows and realizing that I was losing my chest as I leaned out, I decided to save my pennies and make an appointment for myself with the best doctor I could find in my area—it was my birthday present to me. I expressed to my doctor that I was involved in weight lifting and fitness competitions that involved gymnastics so that he was aware of my needs. He recommended that I go under the muscle, through the nipple, and go slightly fuller (with silicone implants) than I had planned, as they would shrink some after the surgery swelling went down. I ended up going with saline instead of silicone simply because I felt it was safer, but he was adamant that silicone was safe.

At that time I had finished my last show for the year and was planning on enjoying the holidays and not worrying too much about training. Sometime in late November or early December I started doing easy cardio once again and by January

(continued on page 114)

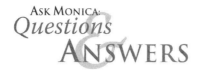
of 1994 I was lifting light weights again. The feeling was strange, and it took some time to regain all of my flexibility, but in no time I was back to practicing my routines for Fitness. I competed in June of '94 with no problems and since then have not had one issue or regret. Just because it has been asked by many people, my breasts still feel natural and soft . . . well, as natural as possible. I have not spent much time massaging them or moving them around, but I have continued to keep stretching for flexibility.

I have and will continue to encourage women to have augmentation if they so desire. Of course I highly suggest that one finds a reputable doctor and do some research on his/her prior patients. I also recommend getting the implant under the muscle, mostly because it makes sense to have a muscle holding the implant in place—not just skin and some breast tissue. Also, if you are going to be competing or leaning down, there is less of chance of "rippling" from the bag. If you do decide on surgery, be sure to give yourself plenty of time to recover and have someone with you for the first week to make sure you do not do any lifting, pulling, or pushing.

Please know that by no means am I saying that a woman has to have implants or needs them to feel good about herself. I am simply trying my best to cover all the different questions I have been asked over the years, and this has been brought to my attention time and again.

Q *I am new to the scene and am curious about competing in Figure or Fitness. Can you please give me some pointers to get started?*

A After making the decision to compete in Fitness or Figure, you will need to map out a program leading up to the date of the contest. If you have never competed before, I suggest giving yourself at least six months to prepare for Figure and longer for Fitness, depending on your background in dance and gymnastics with respect to perfecting a fitness routine.

Fortunately for those of you who are just getting started in the competition field, you have the choice of competing first in Figure and then moving to Fitness at a later date. When I started competing, there was only Fitness, and I *had* to be able to perform a fitness routine! If you are hoping to compete in Fitness, I suggest doing a figure contest first to familiarize yourself with the physique portion. Then you can tackle the routine portion knowing you already have half of it figured out!

So let's take it from a Figure standpoint only. First on the list is to do some research and find a nutritionist in your area who has experience preparing athletes for contests. If you cannot find one in your area, there are some who do online/phone consulting. The nutritionist I use is Kim Oddo (www.bodybyo.com). In my opinion, he is the best and he works with hundreds of athletes all over the country.

Once you establish a relationship with your nutritionist, you will need to have some photos shot of your body in its present condition. You will give these to your nutritionist for the dreaded critique phase where he or she will map out your nutrition plan, training and cardio program, and any supplementation that you may need. Most likely you will need to have your body fat and weight recorded for an accurate body composition analysis.

(continued on page 116)

Your nutritionist will help you plan each week prior to your show and will make sure you are staying on track. Of course, you will have to do your homework if you want the plan to be successful!

There are other things to consider in figure competition, such as contest stage suits, stage shoes, hair and makeup, jewelry, tanning and tanning products, nails and toenails, and skin care for your face and body. By contest time, everything has to be put together and ready to go so that you do not forget anything while you are on your strict diet. Be sure to write down anything important; this will make preparing for your next show slightly easier should you become addicted to competing.

Reading magazines such as *Oxygen, Muscle & Fitness,* and *Muscle & Fitness Hers*, as well as attending local fitness or figure competitions will help you visualize yourself on stage and become familiar with the procedures.

Take plenty of photos from week to week to see your progress. You will not see the slight changes when you look at yourself in the mirror every day, but the photos don't lie!

Attending fitness/figure camps will help you learn from the veterans. If you are interested, I host the F.E.M. Camp and teach training techniques, nutrition, stage poise and presentation, makeup for stage and photos, and participants actually take part in a real photo shoot. To find details and dates for the F.E.M. Camp, log onto www.monicabrant.com and click on MB Fitness Events.

GLOSSARY

CARB: Carb is short for carbohydrate, the main energy source in foods like fruits, vegetables, grains, and sugar.

CARDIO: Cardio is short for cardiovascular exercise, which means aerobic exercise that involves major muscles, such as those found in your legs, and elevates your heart rate. Cardio can include walking, running, cycling, doing an elliptical machine or doing an aerobics class at the gym.

FREQUENCY: How often you do something is known as frequency. For example, your training frequency might be going to the gym three times per week.

INTENSITY: Intensity is a measure of how hard you work. This is sometimes described as working on a 1-10 scale, 10 being hardest.

REP: Rep is short for repetition, which is the act of moving through a complete range of motion one time. For example, one "rep" of a biceps curl would consist of moving the weight up toward your chest then back down again toward your legs.

SET: A set is a given number of repetitions. For example, you might do 10 repetitions of a leg extension and that would equal one set. If you do three sets, that means you do 10 repetitions, rest, do another 10, rest, and finish with your final set of 10 repetitions. A set usually consists of 10 to 20 repetitions. You'll most often perform one to three sets of an exercise.

SMITH MACHINE: The Smith machine is a machine at the gym with a free-weight bar attached to a track that allows it to move straight up and down. You can load the bar with weight plates and then perform many exercises, such as squats, using the machine to help keep your form correct.

SPLIT: Also known as a training split, this is a way to divide your body up so you are not lifting weights for your entire body each time you train. For example, you might do a three-day training split in which you train legs once, chest and triceps once, and back and biceps once.

SPOTTER: A spotter is someone that assists you with the last few reps of any given exercise. For example, your spotter can help lift you once your back starts to fatigue in pull-ups.

DREAM! DESIRE! FOCUS! DISCIPLINE! DEDICATE!

Ladies! These ARE the keys to success and hopefully, after reading this book, you have come to realize that you are not alone in your quests, whether they be for a better physique or just to become healthier—and there is absolutely nothing wrong with wanting these things for yourself.

Achieving these dreams can be as easy as constantly and diligently streaming day-to-day living practices together effectively and efficiently to ensure your proper nutrition, exercise, and emotional balance is intact!

Be strong in your plan of action and make it happen! Don't worry about failure; as long as you are giving it your all, you have nothing to fear. Learn to work with what God gave you as a system—it works! I promise. Remember it will be solely up to you to figure out exactly what system you have been given.

As my original mentor, Marla Duncan, says, "Never underestimate the power of the human body; it is an incredible machine that you can mold and shape into your reality!"

I know you have dreams. Please don't let anyone or anything dictate what your limitations are or should be when it comes to achieving those dreams! Only you can make them happen, so what are you waiting for?

Be sure to associate yourself with positive people who have similar goals and interests as your own. Having a close network of people like this can be a huge source of motivation.

Also, do not forget to enjoy the ride to becoming healthier and fitter. Do not be in a rush. Remember: The turtle won the race! Keep in mind that God blessed each of us with only one body, so be patient and loving to it and nurture it with great care!

All my best wishes for lots and lots of success and, as always: Stay fit, love life, and God bless you!

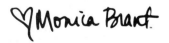